THE SEARCH

THE SEARCH

THE SEARCH

THE LIFE OF A MOUNTAIN RESCUE SEARCH DOG TEAM

PAUL BESLEY

Vertebrate Publishing, Sheffield
www.adventurebooks.com

THE SEARCH

Paul Besley

First published in 2024 by Vertebrate Publishing.

VERTEBRATE PUBLISHING, Omega Court, 352 Cemetery Road, Sheffield S11 8FT, United Kingdom. *www.adventurebooks.com*

A CIP catalogue record for this book is available from the British Library.

ISBN: 978-1-83981-241-5 (Paperback)

ISBN: 978-1-83981-242-2 (Ebook)

ISBN: 978-1-83981-243-9 (Audiobook)

10 9 8 7 6 5 4 3 2 1

Edited by Helen Parry, cover design by Jane Beagley.

Vertebrate Publishing is committed to printing on paper from sustainable sources.

MIX
Paper | Supporting
responsible forestry
FSC
www.fsc.org   FSC® C013056

Printed and bound in the UK by TJ Books Limited, Padstow, Cornwall.

CONTENTS

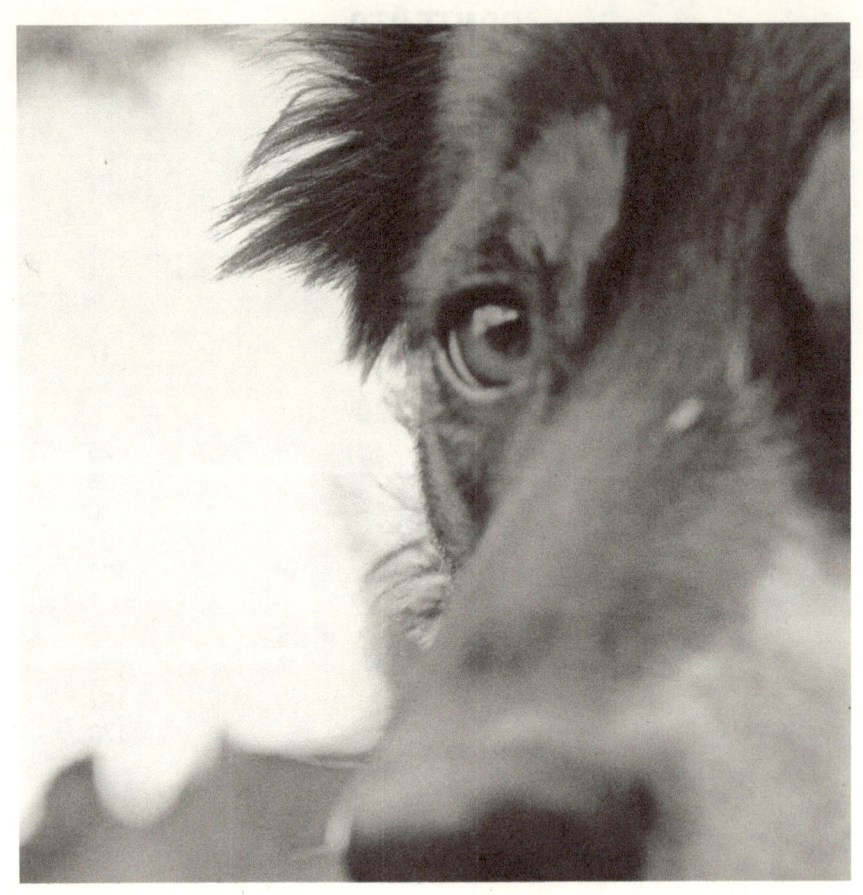

For Scout,
for finding me.

The dog found her in a ditch. She was wet and cold and shivering. The dog barked then ran away.

WINTER 2022

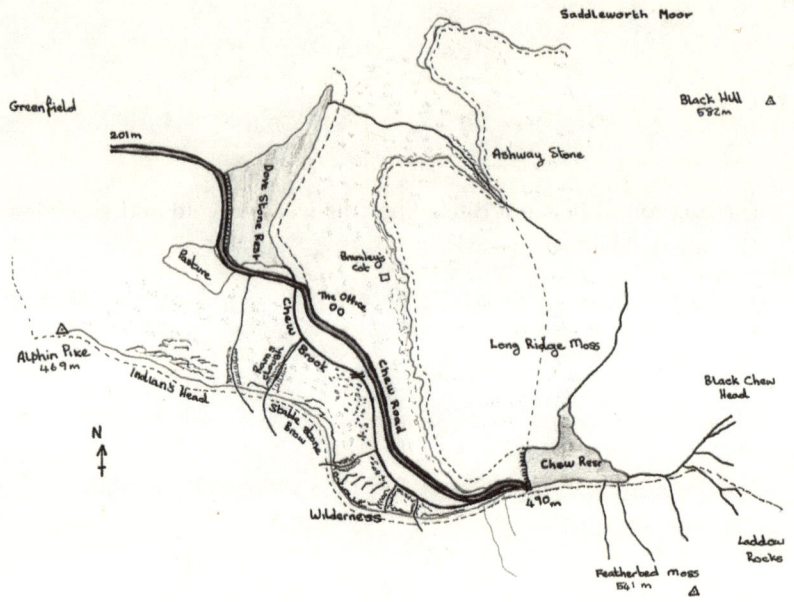

Saddleworth Moor

Greenfield

Black Hill
582m

201m

Ashway Stone

Dove Stone Resr

Bramleys
Cot

Binns

The Office

Long Ridge Moss

Alphin Pike
469m

Chew Brook

Indian's Head

Chew Road

Black Chew
Head

Stable Stone
Brow

Chew Resr

N

470m

Wilderness

Laddow
Rocks

Featherbed moss
541m

PROLOGUE: ON CHEW ROAD

The Chew Road rises 900 feet from the waters in the valley below to the waters in the sky above.

Seasons burnish, without complaint, its thin grey surface sometime tarmac sometime gravel sometime dirt. There is no shade. There are no trees. No birds sing.

The road scratches a line north through peat and rock along the eastern slopes of Chew Valley shadowing the course of bedrock carved by the soft waters of Chew Brook far below. The sun and moon draw their path east to west from blackened gritstone edge to blackened gritstone edge, sliding shadows across a land rarely disturbed by human foot.

People leave narrow streets, escape the factory floor, the school run, the weekly shop, the valley narrowing as the road climbs, people doggedly venturing farther from home further into earth, happy when darkness falls to be safe in the light that comforts them, strengthened for another day.

Most come to live, young sinewy men and women enticed by the thrill of a climb, the feel of rough gritstone grinding knuckles raw, reminded at times that gravity makes no allowance for the audacity of youth. Some know nothing of why the valley has held them, a blanket of darkness falling over a confused, twisted form. Others find a resting place, a view of the setting sun, or home.

The spring equinox wakens coal-blackened rock from a too-long brutal winter, the gritstone blushing with rosettes that bruise through purple and green and brown, lastly bleeding into golden grains of yellow sand and glittering lucid quartz. The waters sparkle amidst emerging soft growth swaying back and forth on a warming breeze.

A westerly brings summer, nudging the valley into colour, swathes of vibrant

green bracken reaching higher than a human, its spread bullying black peat, grey
rock and yellow tussocky grass. Daubes of vivid pink heather dab the hillside
tremoring at the touch of countless bees sizzing across the fragrant blooms. The land
burns often, the sun denying the parched land relief.

Autumn arrives, the landscape easing its descent into a beige middle age, the
peat slick underfoot, hard rain sliding up the valley, dragging the beasts from the
months ahead.

An easterly brings winter raging across the Wilderness, hunkering down
between rock and sky. The roiling black clouds heavy with anger tormenting the
land as they thunder over the long gritstone edge, the valley rumbling as a romance
of black horses pour their harshness into the earth, pounding the ground scattering
beasts and tearing at tussocky peat, thin wisps of blackened bracken twirling in
their long dark manes, the fury lifting to scour the surface of the road until bones
are gnawed.

In summer, it can be a desperate place. In winter, it is hell.

Crouching in Deadman's Lay-by, a small scrap of dirt clawed out of the
moor halfway along the valley, a popular spot for those seeking release, we
stay low, out of the biting wind driving harsh snow into the land and its
inhabitants. Grains of ice blast my cheek raw, the cold piercing through flesh
to bone forcing me further into my hood, for the wind to howl through my
mind laughing. We wait.

Scout chooses his position well: me, his windbreak; his nose pointing
into the disturbance as it blusters past, sampling scents barrelling up the
road. This is his world, his chosen environment of harsh ground in harsh
weather; Border collies are noted for their ability to thrive in inhospitable
extremes. He sits, feet together, glancing occasionally at me, clearing snow
from eyes with a flick of his brow, ears twitching as flakes try to establish a
base. His work jacket offers some protection from the elements; the real
work done by his natural coat and fine downy base layer keeping him warm
and dry. He does not show the cold, does not shiver. Humans are not built
for extremes.

Ice forms on the sleeve of my jacket, pockmarked with effervescence in
the translucent veil. Rime forms on woody heather and yellow blades of
grass. I watch the ice glisten as the winds push its fragility back and forth.
The ice does not fracture.

My radio crackles into life.

'Time for us to go, Scout.' He nuzzles, a snowflake on the tip of his black nose burns my cheek. Ice has fused the join between his coat and fur. He shakes vigorously, jewels fracturing the air with light as he corkscrews free. Across the valley a raven watches. We step off Chew Road …

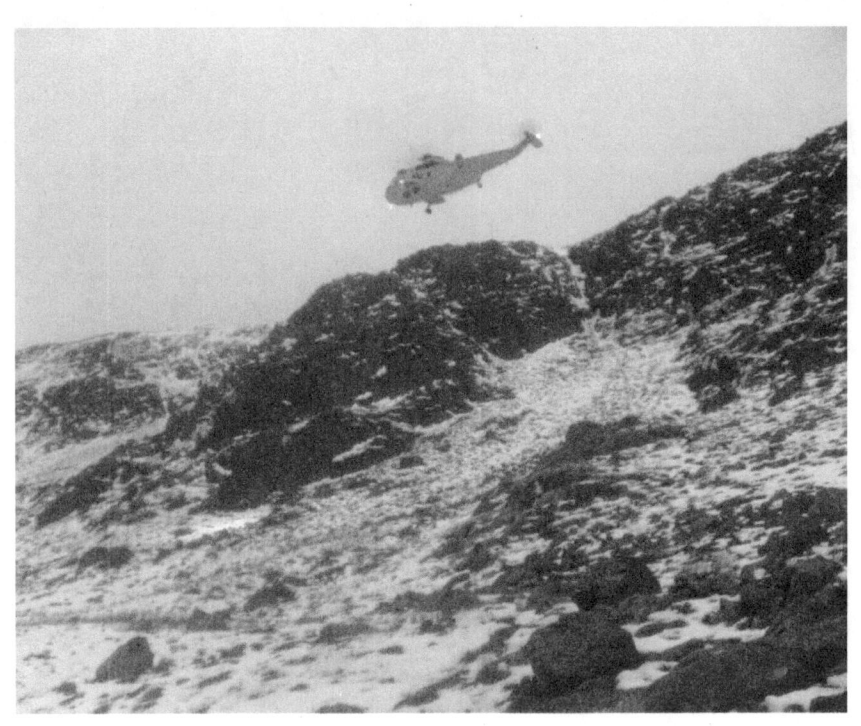

THE FALL

2012

There had been no warmth that day. A cold knife sliced through me folding my body into the howling wind. When the raging quietened I straightened, slowly, and strained eyes for the path to safety. Watching the spindrift scurry across the moor I felt the hollowness of winter carved from my mind and drew further into my shell.

Movement caught my eye. A raven – its blackness blazing against the snow – cast its eye across the moor at me. I smiled. We studied each other as the wind packed snow around our feet and until the bird retreated into the shadows. I stared at the empty space unsure of the encounter. Turning towards the black sky, I moved towards the horizon.

I was tiring from the hours on the hill. My body ached, legs stumbled, feet and poles caught in frozen grass, my mind numbing from effort. The wind pounded my body, never letting up, throwing my balance at every step, the heavy pack slowly leaching out any strength I had. I grumbled at the wind, the words wrenched from my lips and scattered across the moor unheard.

A narrow rivulet cut my line, the running black water at odds in the frozen landscape. The smoothness of the liquid slipped effortlessly through the ice. Clumps of snow drooped down the thin layer of peat grabbing droplets of water to add to ice.

The wind dropped. I let my eyes refocus. Stepped across.

The raven studied the creature's faltering progress, the frailty of it all. The noise the creature made concerned the bird; there was still a thin sheen of daylight, and it

7

feared the noise would bring predators. It sampled the air, feathers riffling, then drew further into the shadows.

The creature looked lost in the vast whiteness, its head bent to the land, the body leaning on long thin limbs struggling to push forwards. With the wind quieting it looked ahead into the darkening sky and moved. The single step, a blast rattling the mountainside, twisting the creature into rock, snow and a red mist scattering in the storm. The raven watched as the creature's head sprang forwards face contorted, then dropped, then vanished; the face not knowing its body was free, a vessel of flesh and bone slithering slowly across the snow, a red band smearing its brief journey. It lay for a moment, then rolled, the silent limp mass slumping over the edge of the crag.

A trailing foot caught a spike of rock, jerking the body, sinew tore, tendons snapped, the mass slamming into the crag face, the sounds of crushing bones and splattering flesh echoing below. A thick strand of blood and tissue dripped, catching on the rock and snow in daubs and pools, a presence drawn from top to bottom, the body following, to the boulder field below. The pack, torn from limbs, jettisoned into the monochrome emptiness, its contents wheeling through space. Behind, the crag strobed as the earth rose, explosions of white and red blasting into the air with each impact of the creature on rock and snow, the silence bouncing and cartwheeling wildly until the whole sorry mess crumpled to a halt in soft snow.

The raven watched the creature's life seep into the gathering cold, then turned from the wind.

Light and cold flood through me, driving me back into the world, not knowing the why or the where of it all, confused, in deep snow. Around, boulders gather like sheep settling in for the night. Below, the distance unknown, a black circular sheet nestled in a white bowl. The lake I was descending to. Perhaps a vague memory of a boot stepping across black running water, from snow to snow, the boot never making it to the second snow. Then blackness.

Light again. A line draws down a cheek, wet, warm and pleasing. I trace the flow with a finger to a hot mushiness; fat red periods drop into the snow, hot blood melting the surface, spreading out through deep red, vermillion, ending in a touch of pink. There's a deep gouge in my head and a big fold of scalp that's squeezed between fingers, tissue, blood and hair tangling with grains of rock and ice. I push a finger into the groove, press, press harder testing the depth, sensing the strangeness of a finger inside my head. There is no pain to see.

There's a valentine dinner at home. An hour should bring the track by the lake, another hour to the car, then home. When I move the lights go out. There's the scratchy image of a boot stepping over water. Then the lights are back on, laid in the snow again, face up to the dying day.

My right side is mangled. The shoulder twisted, chest misshapen, the right foot points the wrong way, a crampon swings freely from the tip of the boot. Movement brings crunching sounds from inside, filling the air with calling, the jagged ends of bone rubbing against one another. I vomit – red, yellow, black, a wrenching pulse screaming out to the coming night, the rancid bile glistening on clothing. My mouth is full of wobbling teeth. My finger pokes again, gingerly, hooking out a slippery mass. Thick gobs of vomit, blood, tissue drip down from bits of teeth, on to raw skin. Thick globules slide off my fingers as I pass the unctuous mess from one hand to the other, trying to keep the flow, mesmerised by the tactile beauty. It's the broken teeth bedded in the roof of the mouth – not the pain in the chest, the wonky foot, or even the finger-sized hole in the head – which pulls the world into focus.

I've left a route map of my day but have little faith that anyone will notice me missing. Sitting in hope in the tightening cold isn't an option; I need help. My phone is in my pack.

I begin to shake; first my legs, then my whole body is in fevered motion. A wave of depression follows, and I begin sobbing uncontrollably, strands of snot, bloody mucus and vomit pour down from my face in vivid braids to pool on the snow. A few moments of this and I've warmed up, the sobbing eases and I regain control enough to scan the boulder field for my pack. I spot it, thirty metres below wedged upside down between two rocks. I have no idea how it got there or how I can get to it.

My left side looks and feels relatively unscathed: a little torn clothing, but no blood and seemingly no broken bones, and the foot points in the correct direction. I reason I can slowly crab my way across the boulders to the pack; it's the best hope of getting help, I'm not going to be doing much else. Inching over to the nearest rock I smear my way to the top on my left-hand side, using my left hand and foot as rack and pinion to jerk me along. My arm goes numb on the cold surface and my hip argues against the deep chill. I try a controlled descent, inching my body, arm outstretched to break any sudden slide into the abyss. My hand touches the snow, then sinks deeper until it touches something solid and stops. My whole weight is now on my freezing fingertips and deadened arm. Suspended upside down

I can't work out what to do next. I settle on a freestyle attempt, letting my mass take me down. It begins well; inch by inch the gap closes as my fingers turn bright red and begin to buckle under the strain. Gravity takes over, again, and I can't hold it so let my body cantilever, the bad leg swinging into rock, snow spraying out, the crampon bouncing like hard rain on a tin roof, the pain powering through my body, then I lose focus and the pain is lost in the darkness that engulfs me.

There is light and an odd upside-down world of cold white and grey. My foot is above me. I can see a crampon spike jammed into my clothing, my mouth tastes metallic, pins and needles flash along my arm, my fingers burn. The lunacy of the descent comes back to me. One more push with my good leg and everything collapses on top of me and it's back to the darkness.

The light is back. I realise I am losing chunks of time; the sky always seems darker after the light is switched back on. I reason I must be drifting in and out of consciousness. That touches my fear.

Shuffling up against a rock, I concentrate on getting my breathing under control, staring at a wide red stripe running down the boulder, marking my descent into the Eton mess of my landing zone. Finely carved crosses in the snow jump up at me. A raven, springing between boulders, marking a way to my pack. I hope. Am I hallucinating or mad?

Crabbing my way forwards – grab-pull-push-repeat, five repetitions then rest and count to one hundred, then go again – I make progress. It's hard work; the downward slopes have me tensing, hampering my breathing. To get a rhythm I pick a soundtrack: 'Another One Bites the Dust' by Queen seems appropriate, and I time my movement to the beat. Thump thump thump of the baseline forming the punctuation of my crabbing grab and push, then I'm there, my hand on the pack and a smile on my face, my body resting in triumph, breathing harshly, feeling the sweat chilling skin and bone.

Behind me there's a shallow run made by my body; a red stripe winds its way between rocks. The blood shouts. All that blood. I pull a bandage out of the kit. Wrapping it around my head with only one useful hand and arm gives me a boost and I begin to think I might get out of this.

I keep my eyes closed, please be there. When I feel the yellow light, I see four bars steady, breathe. I enter a warm world of calm voices. I rattle off my injuries. Slow down. Scalp peeled back, hole in my head, shoulder and chest misshapen, pain, foot pointing in the wrong direction, lots of blood, getting cold, losing consciousness. Yes, I'm on my own. I'm on a mountainside near Coniston. It's getting dark. The voice tells me help is on its way. I whisper 'OK.' The voice says it will call me back.

I feel small and utterly alone, sat staring at the fading land until the cold grips me and I snap back into the present and pull my survival gear out of the pack. The big orange bag doesn't fare well, crampons slice the thick plastic; somehow, I get it around me to stop the wet snow from seeping any further into clothing. I put all my clothes on, in any order, anything to preserve heat. Tea from my flask helps and I use the little I have to wash down the last piece of fruit cake, the crumb mixing with bits of broken teeth and strands of tissue that I poke free to ease the food's journey. I worry about my exact location.

The small yellow square beams at me. It's the voice wanting to know how I'm doing, and what I have been up to, like we've just met down the pub. I go over my actions, wanting the voice to stay with me. It asks for a grid reference. I'm so eager to please I don't think about any difficulty, dig out my map and compass and perform a resection – a resection for pity's sake – quickly as the light is fading fast. I plot three bearings then draw the lines to produce the small triangle of a cocked hat on my map. My position is somewhere in there, an eight-figure grid reference. I give these to the voice, but confidence fails me, and I ask the voice to wait while I repeat the whole process, ending up with a smaller hat in the same place. I give the voice a ten-figure grid reference, placing me in a one-metre square, below Raven Tor and above Levers Water. The voice gasps and I can hear a smile. Redemption.

I worry that rescuers won't see me so put my head torch on, the band catching the groove in my head, twisting it to one side. Consciousness drifts, half light and half sound. I hold conversations, sleep, wake to Alison asking what time I will be home. I see a family, all in red, walking; they tell me they are walking up to me, and I think this is madness, why would anyone want to be out on a night like this. Everything is dark now. There is no definition, my world squeezed down to a ten-figure-grid-reference square metre of snow and rock and the flickering shadows. I am so tired that all I want to do is rest.

In the cocoon of my warm world someone is drumming. A bell chimes. An animal circles around me barking into my face, its hot breath pleasing me. A roaring wind pushes me into the earth and out of the darkness into a vast white light that catches swirling snow and holds me in a pool of noise and movement flickering high above. Shadows rage in between the rocks and the snow. The lake has gone. The white bowl too. All that exists is light and sound. I release myself into the light, tears whipping off my face as shapes loom larger out of the black emptiness that holds the light.

A shadow. I move, trying to get back into the life-giving pool, but a hand stops me, gently presses my arm and a voice says, 'You're safe now.'

One week later I'm home, trying to make my foot go over the doorstep so I can get in the house. The nerve connections just aren't there and, try as I might, I cannot get my leg to lift those few inches. It's all very unsettling. Over the coming weeks I move from the settee, on hands and knees, upstairs to bed. Each day Alison brings me a plate of sandwiches, a bag of crisps and a Tunnock's, then leaves for work. The food is gone by mid-morning. Other than urinating I have been unable to make use of the toilet for three weeks. In desperation I resort to using a spoon and dig myself free; the relief is unimaginable, so good that I relive the delicious moment over and over in my mind.

At night I sleep with a cocktail of painkillers my mind is happy to use. A scratchy reel of light and dark that breaks my sleep gradually coalesces into the snow and rock of the crag face I hurtled down. When I wake, covered in sweat, my traumatised mind trying to grab hold of the sense of it all, there is nothing but confusion. To exorcise this ghost, Alison and I head back in July to walk the route again. When we reach the small brook, I step over it and wait. Nothing comes, my memory remains steadfastly closed to the moments between that step and consciousness at the foot of Raven Tor.

I've always seen the importance of giving back. When I assumed I would not be reported missing, I was wrong. I was reported missing at the exact time I was supposed to have returned. The fact that a rescue operation was already in progress was irrelevant. I sent a letter of thanks to the manager at Holly How youth hostel, and his CEO; later that year he received a reward for that night. The nurses and surgeon in the hospital received chocolates and a card of thanks. I sent a donation to the Coniston Mountain Rescue Team who saved me along with a letter of thanks. The treasurer phoned me a few days later to thank me. He told me there were seventeen people and a dog involved on the ground that winter night. That made me feel terrible; I apologised for all the fuss I had created, disturbing people's night.

'No, no,' he said, 'you were a proper rescue, you had really stuffed yourself, we all had a fantastic time.' Thank you seemed insignificant.

They reckon that, after a trauma, people either spend the rest of their life on the settee watching TV or become more extreme in the thing that nearly killed them. Happily, for me, it's the latter. I explore remote places, tethered by a satellite tracker to give Alison ease of mind. As my body heals, my mind plays catch-up. Self-belief has always been an issue, but my survival has shifted the ground – if the worst nearly happened, there's nothing to fear. It's a moment that begins unpicking the knots from decades of conditioning.

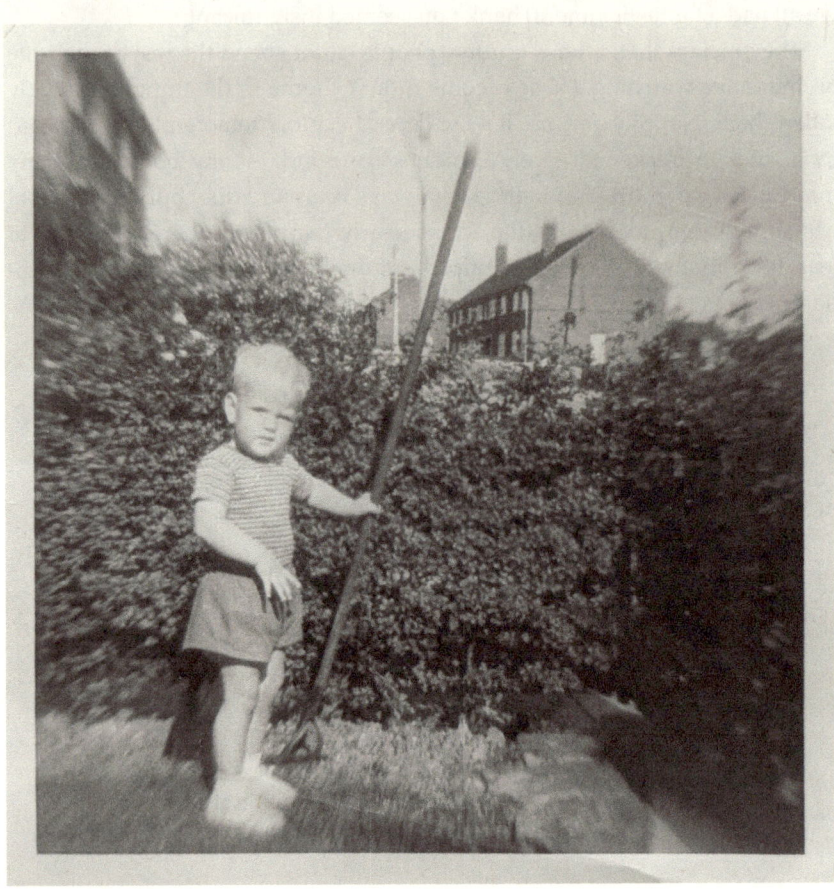

THE ANOMALY

THE ANOMALY

1959-2012

If I'd had the confidence to say what kind of life I wanted things may have been different. But I didn't. And it wasn't.

Dad's mood was the gravity we danced around: Mum, older brother, and me. At any moment the world could shrink tight, the light punched out as fists landed from all angles, toes found soft spaces under ribs, the maniacal look on that red face, gorged with pleasure, the flecks of white spittle flying from clenched teeth as the rage took control and I'd see the whiteness of the knuckles as they filled the view, then be lost in the explosion of pain, and I knew, I just knew, he didn't see me. Always on the stairs away from neighbours' telling ears and eyes, clawing my way up, pulling at threads of carpet fearful I'd tear holes in the pattern, trying not to scream, the tears stinging, legs grabbed and twisted, my head thumping down each step for more beating. And I'd try not to make a sound because that got the beating beaten in more. Mum sat in the room, telly turned high, a chocolate digestive to dunk in tea, the Marks and Spencer cup and saucer balanced on the arm of the chair, the antimacassar removed for cleanliness. My older brother in his bedroom, door closed. I'd tell school I got into a fight; getting the look of contempt and disgust I learned to keep the truth of it all deep inside.

I didn't like school and was glad to leave, surprising most with reasonable grades. Dad looked at the offers sat at the table in the dining room of the council house we lived in. He feared one day losing his job and home, his own childhood reaching into our lives today. Now, I realise that in his world everything was a risk, everything. He never owed money; we went without. A week in Blackpool each year, all in one bedroom, the smell of fried bread and fatty bacon permeating every corner of the boarding house

17

that was so far away from the sea it could have almost been inland. Wet beds staving off unwanted fumblings; the shame of rubber sheets. Constant rain.

With tea done, Mum washing the pots, older brother in his bedroom, I stood by the table. A degree in English or the steel mill. The steel mill was my place Dad said, a job for life. That was it. A lifetime passed in a moment. I was sixteen. The steel mill closed nine years later.

I loved the mill. It was dirty and dangerous and had a family that looked after me. The canteen ladies would give me extra bacon, another slice of toast, build me up for a man's world. Some looked at me with pained eyes, ask if I was my dad's kid, reach across and give me a peck on the cheek and a squeeze, then push me away, no payment required. The men teased: KJ, one of the labourers, gave me a love bite when they found out I had a girl-friend; the others holding me down, he took his yellow teeth out, washed them in cold tea, then sucked away. They watched over me, kept me out of flying cobbles of red-hot steel streaking through the air, showed me where to stand on the furnace roof so that if it went in, I could jump away from the bubbling molten steel two feet below. Taught me craftsmanship, how to make pipe joints in copper, leather and asbestos, everything neat. How to bend pipes with sand, how to weld hanging upside down by my feet. Took me home for dinner. Took me to the pub. I was part of a community and, for the first time, felt wanted.

The mill was full of men who weren't afraid to step forward, looking out for each other. Red was one. A character that stood out for all the wrong reasons, while quietly standing for all the right ones. Famous for never washing, you smelled him before you saw him; he wore the same clothes day in day out, year in year out, drank antiseptic neat from the bottle, always had a cigarette burning. He lived with two prostitutes, hot-bedding the only bed in the house. And he kept an eye on me. When they started to close the mills, Red offered to take my place, said the future, whatever it was, was for the young. It didn't come to that, but I never forgot his kind-ness. Years later I'd stand him and the girls a round whenever I caught them in a pub. The girls would ask me if I wanted to head home and I'd blush and make my excuses and they'd give me a peck on the cheek, whisper some ecstasy in my ear while a hand slid down and brought me to life.

Use giant machines to move hot metal around at speed and someone, evetually, will get hurt. Steel mills were populated by men with bits miss-ing, some visible, most hidden behind burning eyes. The pubs were inhabited by those that held the long waking hours together with alcohol. I'd found a home.

We'd spend our days drifting between the steel mill and the pub. It once must have seen good days but was now inhabited by men in greasy overalls, arguments, broken furniture, and a floor that was a patchwork of faded oilcloth and grease-stained boards. The pub smelt of stale beer, rotting plaster, and the metallic tang of steel slag. An atmosphere of nervous depression lived at the bottom of every pint. I sat and watched as a regular chatted up the landlady while her husband drank away the meagre profits. I had a sense it wouldn't last.

At weekends we'd head into town, everyone in their finery, the men in handmade suits, crisp shirts and polished shoes. The girls striving to be Olivia Newton-John, the big hair with enough hairspray to punch a hole in the atmosphere. We'd begin with a crawl through the pubs, pacing our drinks, timing each arrival for the free food, mini Yorkshire puddings with rabbit gravy, ham sandwiches, tripe and vinegar, bag and chitlins. At closing we'd drift across to one of the clubs, a nod to Harry on the door in his tux, his sweat towel left in the finishing mill. Two a.m. we'd have the last dance, gazing into the eyes of a girl we'd just met, while 10cc spun out, 'I'm Not in Love'. If the weather was good, we'd walk home, calling at Gordon's single decker abandoned on waste ground under the railway arches. The windows would be steamed up, the inside full of couples polishing off big plates of fried food, eggs swimming in pools of yellow fat, sausages popping at the first stab, the spray consigning another tie to the bin. Gordon stood where the back seat should have been wheeling several pans across burning hobs. A big tea urn puttered steam into the tightening space. He'd shout out orders holding a plate of food in one hand, a mug of tea in the other and a Park Drive bringing tears to his eyes, a Hogarthian figure of unhygienic magnificence. Hands would grab plates, pass them over heads until they reached whoever could remember their order. A sugar bowl would be needed and eventually appear. All this amid a cacophony of conversation and squeals of gritty laughter; girls talked about boys and boys slid furtive glances. Cigarettes would send up smoke to mix with the steam so you couldn't tell one from the other in the light that escaped from the nicotine-coated bulbs. On your way out, the floor crackling and crunching as your new shoes slid through the grease, sugar and tab ends, you'd catch a girl's eye, put her in the memory. Life was simple and good.

On rest days I'd explore the high hills. I liked the solitude of the landscape, its permanence. I took photos and fancied being a photographer, but Dad said I needed to know my place, so I sold my gear and alcohol eased further into the void. I walked and boozed and hung on to resentments, polishing them until the hatred shone bright. The landscape faded into the background and my mind closed to any future. Two years later Dad was dead, ravaged by cancer. A year after, my long-term relationship ended. She said all I was interested in was sex and drink. I'd no template of love to follow so she was probably right, though she omitted to tell me about the new man. We'd just bought a house. I retreated into its walls, living off take-away food and beer, a mound of copper coins piling up on the kitchen floor my one achievement. There was no heating and no furniture. It was damp and miserable. Sometimes I'd sleep in a park for a few days, just for a change. I wasn't doing good.

I got married. Five months later she was holed up in the spare room with a baby. I headed to the pub.

After the steel mill closed the town descended into denial. Loan sharks moved in, followed by drugs, and begging. There's a new office block where the pub stood; outside, a line of shiny BMWs on shiny black tarmac, no doubt deep carpets and comfy chairs inside. It will be missing the characters and that sense of belonging. Without the mill we all slowly drifted apart. I heard the lad chatting up the landlady had married her daughter and that Red had died. One Christmas I saw the two girls in a pub. They gave me a sorrowful smile. I put some money behind the bar for them and raised a glass to us all.

I got a job selling engineering parts and nailed myself to a cross every day. Fearing rejection, I spent my day hiding in lay-bys and drinking, eventually reaching home to another argument. It wasn't a successful sales technique. I knew the walls were closing in. By my mid-twenties I'd got a family, a mortgage, a barely secure job and a major drink problem. It all came crashing down. I came out of a two-week blackout to find people staring at me and someone with blood on their face. I knew then if I was to have any sort of life, I couldn't mix me and drink. It wasn't my friend.

I managed to find people who were willing to show me a path to a way of living without alcohol and I held on for all I was worth. They were trying to find a life they could fit into. Most had been through several lives; like at the steel mill there were characters that had spent too much time in the dark. I gravitated to those shadows. The one-eyed tattooed armed bank robber (failed), hiding from his former gang. The army major who got hammered on duty, thought the Russians were invading and had to be pulled away from the button. We'd all found our way through the dark, pushed the door open and decided to stay and see what happened. These days, the major raises pigs in Thailand where he's clocked up over five decades without a drink and says he's happy. The bank robber disappeared one night. I heard a rumour he was part of the foundations of a London office block. I hope he was still sober.

I became good at selling. As sobriety grew so did my career and so did the chasm back home. Finally, I called it a day. I walked away with my whole life in two black bin bags. I was forty years old.

I headed back to the hills, battered by four decades of a life I seemed ill equipped for. I walked and raged against the world. My anchors began to break loose dragging at my confidence. I saw myself unhappy and disembodied from life. Stepping off the corporate treadmill I ground out a living in low-paid jobs, bit my tongue and hoped for something to happen. I sat with friends, talked through the disjointed bits and pieces of a life, trying to see how it all hung together. They listened and I listened; we drank lots of tea.

One day I met Alison. She was, truth be told, everything that terrified me about a woman: stunningly beautiful, highly intelligent, and inhabited a world of art that I had no experience of. It took me eight weeks to pluck up the courage to ask her on a date. We married three years later.

Alison gave me space to explore what I wanted from life. Like me, she had a love of mountains, and dogs. Holidays and weekends were filled with time on summits and under stars. I gained mountain skills, had winter adventures, gradually extended my level of knowledge and expertise.

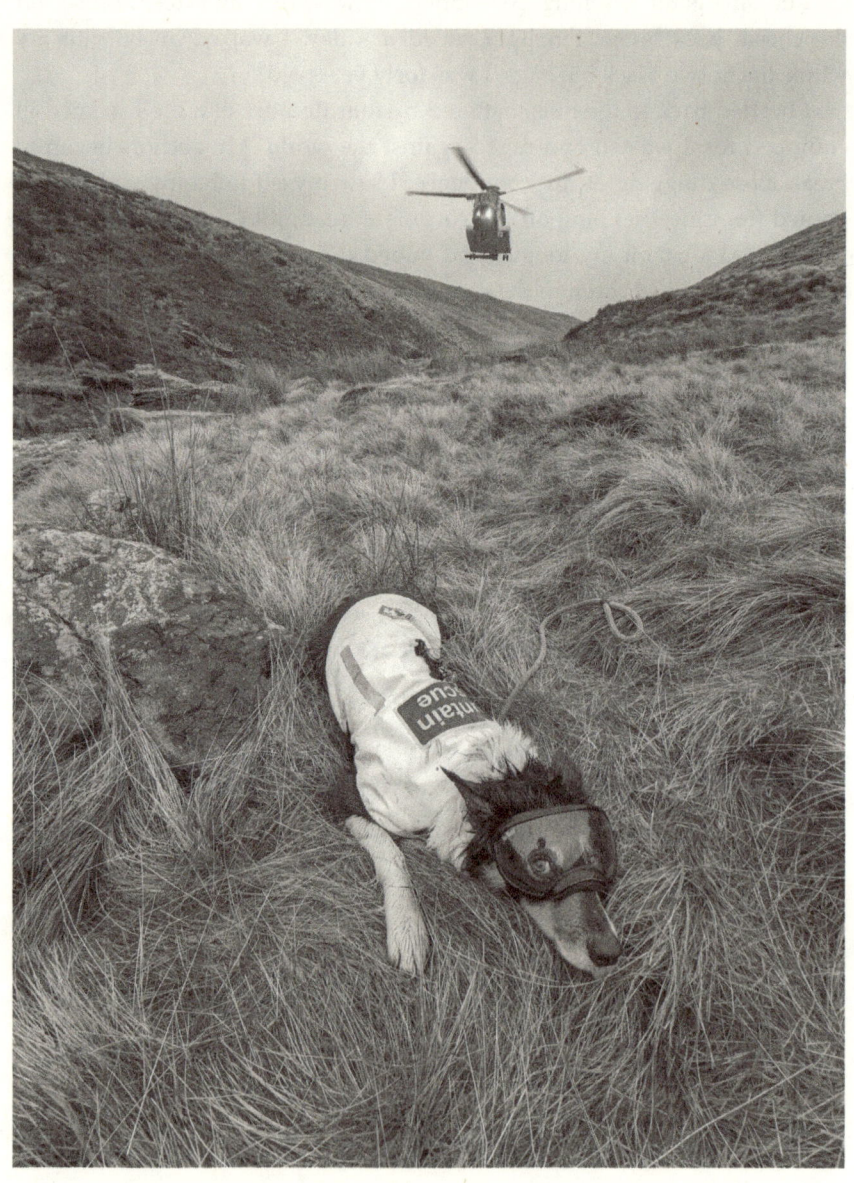

THE SEARCH

2013

Twenty-four of us, nervous strangers, stand in a circle outside a lonely farmhouse in the Pennines, waiting to be interviewed, sifted and selected to train as a member of a mountain rescue team. By the time we are full team members, twelve months later, there will be three of us left standing.

Joining a Peak District mountain rescue team is a way of paying back for my rescue in the Lake District. Gratitude is something I think is important. Training was a daunting process, all those ropes, advanced first aid, fitness. With the shape of my body, I knew I would never be a crag rat plucking people off a rock face, or a fell runner in a snatch squad flying across the moors to rescue some damsel in distress. I was quite happy being a donkey, carrying gear up to a casualty location, carrying it back down, carrying a casualty on a stretcher, manning the radio. I was good at navigation; finding a location was never an issue, and I liked to set up exercises on the moor at night for others to practise their navigation skills. I slotted into my place and trudged up hills.

With my background in engineering I managed the team's buildings, making sure everything was up to scratch, fitting it out to make life easier. I took on the role of social media and press. With the number of call-outs rising, it was important that we raise the money to keep the team operational – pumping out stories of call-outs and training was the easiest way to reach as many people as possible.

Call-outs are the core of what any team member will do. Members are on call every minute of every day of every year and will attend if they are able to. The days of ringing round for volunteers are long gone, now a text message sends us out of the door to a road head where we are briefed, tasked and deployed. We can be out for a few minutes – false alarms, the casualty found by the public. Or hours, sometimes days, no matter the weather or the terrain. Many call-outs come in the early hours before dawn. Partners wait, unsure whether to raise the alarm for people who have failed to return.

Training replicates call-outs, refining skills, familiarising with new equipment. They happen once a week for a few hours at night, sometimes a whole night, or day. It isn't testing, but training, learning what we can do and need to do better.

The testing of the core skills of crag rescue, search and navigation, required by all team members to stay on the call-out list, happens every year. Crag rescue and navigation seem to be the most feared. My favourite is the navigation test. The team will also add fitness in later years, the age profile of team members continuing to head north.

Team members are unpaid volunteers; bizarrely, we used to have to pay to be in a team. There are no expenses for fuel, vehicles or personal kit. With the lost evenings at home, the cancelled days out, the numerous dinners put in the oven or the dog, the work can put a huge strain on home life. Partners and family are the unsung heroes of mountain rescue, aiding a team member to help strangers in distress.

I've navigated for dog handlers on call-outs and find the relationships with their dogs and the work they do fascinating. There are two handlers in my own team who I gravitate to, seeing the intricacies of dog management: handler and dog working together away from the rest of the team, seeking out a casualty purely by scent. It's a dark art straight out of wizardry, and a role I'm becoming more and more attracted to.

I spend days being a dogsbody (body), hiding out on moors and mountains in all weathers for search dogs to find me in training exercises. I get to know handlers and other dogsbodies, noting who seems to know what they are doing. I observe which dogs are better at handling terrain and weather.

The most ubiquitous search dogs are Border collies, perfect for the work, especially if they come from sheep farming stock. Spaniels are favoured by those, it is fair to say, who are super fit or don't realise they have to be. Labradors and retrievers have their supporters, as do German shepherds, the original search dog that was introduced into British mountain rescue by Hamish MacInnes. I favour a Border collie; I like their nature, their joy on the hill, the character they show. All the good handlers I know have a Border collie.

Search dogs are trained separately to the team and more frequently, twice a week, and a whole weekend every month somewhere in Britain. As well as training with the team and attending non-dog call-outs it's a huge personal commitment, so the sponsorship of the team, and more importantly support from partner and family, are required. After two years as a donkey, my team – and Alison – give me the go ahead and I'm accepted to train to be a search dog handler.

All I need now is a dog.

2016

A dog handler has told me about a farmer in the Lake District who breeds working Border collies, many of whom have found their way into mountain rescue as air-scenting search dogs.

This brings us speeding across the Pennines, tyres thrumming on tarmac as we pass underneath the Pennine Way and punch out into the grey skies of Lancashire.

The air in the car is dense, trapping Alison and I between the windscreen and the seats. She chooses words carefully, keeping the conversation light, focusing on the excitement of a puppy coming into our home, being part of our family; her toes feel their way over the eggshells.

We come from different worlds. Me: corporate, industry, comprehensive, council house. Alison: the arts, public school, exotic places. It's why our relationship works. But I have so many hang-ups, such a thin skin, that some days Alison is an adult with a man-sized five-year-old. Anything can press my buttons and there's no consistency, except the days of silent sulks that always follow. At first it had drawn her down: fearing she'd be overwhelmed, she talked to friends, established her own terms for life and stayed. There was good, good that far outweighed the bad. *I knew.* Knew that I was capable of extreme kindnesses and unbelievable cruelties and knew how Alison saw that weighed on me.

When I talked about training to be a search dog handler, she'd asked, tentatively choosing her moment, would I be able to hold it all, or would it crush me? She'd used the word 'endeavour' – the word chosen long before in that curt letter from the search dog training committee. 'We wish you every success in your endeavour,' making it sound like some great adventure of uncertain success. Alison thought the word wise. Someone had walked the path before.

She'd worried. Knew I didn't handle people well, had witnessed my volcanic outbursts, and tried to reach me. I'd spat words, lost in my own darkness, white flecks of spittle spattering from snarling lips. Eventually it would pass, the madness I called it, dissipating until quietness settled upon me, and at last, I would be able to tell her what had happened, how some perceived slight had sent me spiralling into the darkest corner of my mind. Maybe it was the fall, the crack on the head. Maybe it was other stuff long ago. The loving would follow, and we would begin again the cycle of our days, forever watchful of the broken eggs. None of this bode well, we both knew that.

I don't have a good framework for life. It's all I have, though I fight against it. In opening up to Alison, I realise I miss the mentors from the steel mill teaching me about life. That's what I need. I'm so lost in thought that I don't feel Alison reach out until she squeezes my hand, says all will be well, many have done this, relax and enjoy it. My shoulders drop and the grip on the wheel eases, rounded hills appear, I see and feel me and a dog walking across the tops. We slide off the motorway and head west winding through mountains holding the sky, the roads narrowing.

The farmhouse stands at a crossroads, the roads lined with oak and birch, a thin verge separating the tarmac from a drainage ditch. The corners of the house are red stone, in between a mix of flint and granite shards mixed with oatmeal mortar. Through the gate, a scree turning circle with a fountain in the centre, beyond, a large blue door under a stained-glass light. We drive in and wait, unsure if this is the right farm or the right entrance. Do people in the countryside use the front door or back? I get out to a cold wind trying not to look like a townie or be afraid of the barking on the other side of the door. Locks turn, the door wrenches open to reveal a flame-haired woman in a blue woolly jumper, jeans and purple wellingtons, the daughter. 'Entrance is round in the yard.' I start back to the car in embarrassment, but she calls us through. We pass down a hallway stuffed with paintings, mirrors and bric-a-brac into a large kitchen to face a piece of solid Victorian furniture with wispy sandy hair, a ruddy face and hands so large that I think he is wearing thick work gloves.

The daughter slips out and we sit with my nerves. The farmer runs through my credentials. What work do I do? My CV is met with ambivalence. Where do we live? A city. Northern. Near a national park. Minutes from it. I keep laying down facts in the hope that more really is more, but I sense my credibility and confidence ebbing during the interview. Do we have dogs now? I sit up, having slumped under the weight of interrogation. Firmer ground now. Two Bedlington Lakeland terriers, I emphasise the Bedlington and overemphasise the Lakeland. Are they working dogs? Fingers stabbing upwards to clench shut around the answer. No, I reply softly. Fingers fold. The ground shifts again, my position edging towards precarious. Perhaps my honesty disarms him as he seems unsure of my suitability. Honest, yes. But a dog handler? I think about Dad. I sit and smile at the unsmiling face. We sit in silence.

The room fills with frigid air scouring the tiled floor, running round the room to meet the daughter in the doorway. In the palm of her hand a tiny bundle of black, white and tan. Alison gasps. A tricolour, not a black and white. I'd had visions of being out on the hill with a proper collie, like other handlers. The daughter retreats behind the farmer holding the puppy close. The farmer watches me. Another 'aw' from Alison. I can feel her wanting to hold the bundle, this pet. What must they be thinking? The daughter whispers soft words to the puppy, steps forward and places the dog in my lap.

He feels so soft. I gently stroke his paws, the pads bright pink and fleshy, the white socks pristine. He smells of puppy and hay. His nose is black, wet and twitching; deep brown eyes watch me. I whisper hello, place a kiss on the white flash in the centre of his forehead.

The daughter kneels before us and tickles the dog's chin. 'What will you call him?'

I whisper soft words, his fur tickling my nose, take a long look into his eyes. Then I fall.

'Scout. His name is Scout.'

One p.m. on April 28th and we're heading south for home, Scout nested in my lap swaddled in a soft shirt steeped in two days of my scent; a new world of smell, colour and sound rush by.

I'd had no shortage of advice from handlers – what dog to get, how to keep it, how to house train – advice as numerous and as diverse as there are breeds. One piece stuck. In the first six months I must ensure the dog bonds with me and only me.

I say to Alison, I don't think it is a good idea she interacts with him, no calling, no feeding and no petting. Her words are broken, pleading. A tear draws a line down her face; I set my face to the road ahead, the journey onwards passing in silence.

At home we introduce Scout to his new brothers, Bedlington twins. Monty, the stoic of the two, sniffs interest until Olly, who is not happy, not happy at all, pulls him back into line. Scout, eight inches high, stands his ground. Olly growls, I growl, Monty drifts between the growls, Alison attempts to keep everything from spinning outwards.

I set up a wire crate in the basement, away from the bustle of the house and inquisitive Monty. It is cool and dark, the crate holding layers of soft bedding and toys, blankets over the outside of the cage to cocoon him in warmth and quiet. This will be his sleeping quarters much to the dismay of Alison who had envisaged a more homely family life. On the first night, after placing him in bed I sit close by peeping through the blankets to find Scout sitting upright, wide awake and waiting to see what happens next. After an hour with no sound, I slip away. As I reach the floor above a high-pitched sweeping wail fills the house and runs out into the street. I ignore it, needing to be firm. By 3 a.m. with not a single break the wail morphs into a tortuous scream. I stare at the ceiling while Alison sends out waves of 'I told you so.' After a week of banshee nights followed by days of glowering neighbours, I bring the crate into the kitchen, tacitly admit defeat and suggest to Alison that it may help if she shares some of the time with Scout, who, sensing Alison is the real centre of the family, plays the cute little puppy. I'm impressed.

During the day we play, getting Scout used to basic obedience work. Tiny treats underpin desired behaviour; sitting on command comes easily. Monty and Olly sense an easy win and join in, so I have three pairs of eyes fixed on my hand, tails wagging furiously, and Scout happy to be part of it all. It is tiring for Scout. He sleeps a lot curling up in his crate, a ball of fluff fast asleep in minutes. It gives us all a break to reflect on the challenges of parenthood. By the third week we're settled into a routine: food, ablutions, play, sleep, and repeat. At night I put him to sleep, and Alison and I sit close by talking softly until a light snore drifts out from the cocoon. We sleep too, Alison happy that she can finally love Scout and her family is whole.

Our mornings are a whirl of activity – Monty and Olly like spinning tops, toenails chattering around the kitchen floor pressuring me for their breakfast. Scout sits in his crate: feet firmly planted together, head high, back straight, still and watchful. I scoop him out with one hand; he feels warm and fat, his pink tummy spreading through my fingers, his pink tongue licking my hand, its roughness sanding away bits of my scent, my code. He wets his nose to transfer the scent while his eyes hold mine. I smile, press my nose into his coat, draw in that puppy aroma, softly repeat, 'Scout, Scout.'

Monty has always had most of the attention; having worked out Scout is staying he's increased efforts to stay in front, cuddles and treats becoming his prime objectives for the day. Olly sits at the end of the kitchen watching, shooting looks at me.

I want Scout to have a firm routine. Building a framework to his day will help him settle as well as allowing me to concentrate on his training. Breakfast at 7 a.m. the first link in this daily chain. I feed him in his crate to prevent fights breaking out with Monty and Olly, getting him to sit before placing the food bowl, embedding in his psyche the reward system we will use for training and life. After a few days he gets the message and sits in anticipation when he sees me going to put food in his bowl; he learns quickly, we both do. I learn I can produce desired behaviour.

After breakfast we go into the garden. For the first two weeks until his inoculation period is complete Scout is confined to home. We work on routine and getting him used to his name and some basic obedience. We've had a warm start to spring – the garden is alive with colour and smell, the season of new beginnings drifting through the air, birds chatter and flit about carrying scraps into hedges. Scout sits on the doorstep unsure what to do. His nose twitches constantly as his senses are bombarded, his head moving sharply when a sound pulls his attention.

Monty and Olly are rooting around in the flower borders, identifying last night's visitors. Scout watches. I watch Scout. I tell him to go and pee. He looks at me, the gaze steady. I can't expect him to instantly understand commands, so I pick him up and take him into the yard, then walk into the garden calling him as I go, my eyes on him, his eyes on me, his body rock still. I crouch down, nearer his eye level, keeping my voice light and inviting. Up he gets and totters forward, the little legs pumping away, the pudgy behind swaying side to side. Everything is ungainly and haphazard, but I am filled with joy as he reaches me and praise him profusely, ruffling his hair, my voice slipping into baby talk. Monty, hearing all the attention, sidles over for his share. Olly sits way off, hackles raised. When Monty realises there are no treats, he wanders off to explore more of the garden. Scout watches him and glances at me. He wants to play with the other two, but he's not sure how. He looks at me, so I lead him in, making clucking noises until he follows, his attention drawn to what Monty and Olly are doing, but staying close to me; the thread that ties us short, his dependence on me total.

Scout pecks the air, his nose tracing the molecules of scent drifting around us. I try to smell what he is smelling: flowers, soil, stone; somewhere bacon is being cooked. There's a sweet, sticky smell wafting over the town from the doughnut factory, floating images of oozing jam and sticky fingers.

Scout takes an interest where Olly has left a calling card, so I guess sugar-coated confectionary isn't his thing.

Monty is amongst the flowers devouring blades of grass and giving Scout sideways glances. Olly is at his regular spot, sniffing where the hedgehog lives. The two have never met, so the scent fascinates him. It's also where our resident frog lives, layers and layers of scent oblivious to my nose but an extensive library to a dog. Olly takes his time to catalogue the scent, spending minutes at each scent pool, sharp breath drawing in the chemical base then stepping back to analyse and ponder, his head cocked to one side testing a hypothesis. Scout watches, his tiny nostrils flaring, his eyes firmly on Olly. Perhaps this is his first step in becoming an air-scenting search and rescue dog?

He meanders through the garden taking a wandering track that delivers him to Olly's scent pool, sticks his nose in here and there, then ambles over to Monty who turns and gives him a thorough inspection. Scout rolls over, feet in the air in submission; Monty pins him and begins to play, the sound of mewing drifting out of the lilies. A yelp stops everything; Olly, watching in agitation as his brother makes his displeasure known. Monty retreats into the flowerbed planting a calling card on the edge of the path. Scout goes over, tests the scent then adds his own details. The thread that binds me and Scout has lengthened. At ten weeks old, Scout is psychologically smart enough and sure enough for any opportunity, thinking through situations as they happen without any input from me.

It has been a good morning. I can see how Scout already works with scent. It must be an explosion of scent after all his time on the farm and it's interesting that the scents he smells are not interfered with by the human confections of doughnuts and bacon. It's clear he knows how to find a scent pool, and what to do with it.

I call his name and all three turn to look. It's just a sound now with no connection to a dog. I try again; this time only Scout turns, but still does not move. I hold out a treat and call; Monty and Olly bound over. Scout follows, his stubby legs and puppy fat tripping itself looking like he's trying to jump and run at the same time. He halts at the step out of the garden; I encourage him on, keeping Monty and Olly at bay with my hand. Finally, Scout tumbles off the step, his body crumpling into a heap of soft loveliness, then scrambles upright, gets his bearings and trots over for his reward. I keep saying his name, imprinting on his mind who he is. Olly growls and I tell him to stop. He sulks. As Scout crunches down on the treat I tell him how clever he is, what a good boy he is. His eyes stay fixed on mine. I give him another treat to increase the pleasure value of the reward and slip a treat to Monty and Olly for being so understanding. 'We can do this,' I tell Scout.

Before acceptance on to the search dog training programme, handler and dog must demonstrate the ability to command and perform a set standard of obedience: walk to heel on and off the lead; perform a recall (return on command); perform a down stop on command; and perform a down stay for ten minutes including five minutes out of sight of the handler.

Following a successful completion of the above, the dog must undertake a field stock test with sheep to the following standard: the dog is recalled through the flock to the handler; the dog to retrieve a toy placed in the centre of the flock; and the dog to remain in a down stay while the flock is repeatedly run past at close range.

If at any time during the test the dog chases sheep the assessment is terminated and recorded as a fail.

On successful completion of these assessments the dog team can progress to the search dog training programme.

Three members from Peak District mountain rescue teams, including me, along with our dogs, begin obedience training today. I name us the First, Second and Third Man. Myself and the Second Man arrived last night. As yet, there is no sign of the Third Man.

The village hall noticeboard is papered with maps, hills and woodland outlined in thick red crayon. Below each, a list of names: dogs left, humans right. Above each listing are the classifications for each training area, stages one, two and three, and operational. At the bottom of the board is *Obedience Class*, no map just the word 'FIELD' in capitals. Scout is on this list, his first mention in orders. I read it over and over, silently forming his name. Opposite Scout, my name under the heading 'Handler.' Capital H.

In a short time, in a field, in a village in Yorkshire we begin our journey. The responsibility, excitement and trepidation layer through me, my mind tumbling through each then cycling back again. I must tell Scout I will not let him down.

He has slept all night in the van, his first time. His crate swaddled in blankets to form a cosy environment, a soft toy in the corner, a van window cracked for fresh air. I guess he can hear the comings and goings, dogs barking good morning to the world as they head for ablutions. Lifting him out of his bed, his paw pads bright and pink reaching out, his coat warm, soft and silky, the smell of sleepy puppy lifting from his body, I stick my nose into all this happiness and murmur my allegiance to him, restate my promise, my eyes closing as the ache washes over me.

We join the procession of dogs and handlers. Scout has never seen so many, never had such a cacophony of new sights, sounds and smells. He zigzags on his lead, his short legs stumbling over the rough track as he tries to collect everything that is happening, me tap dancing around him in fear of treading on him. Handlers stop and coo at him, dogs sniff, the odd one bristles and gets a scolding. Soon we are surrounded by chatter; there are no pretences of being hard mountain people. All that is present is joy at a perfect little dog.

The authenticity test begins. 'Where is Scout from?' I mention the Lake District farmer and Scout's operational half-brother and his handler. A murmur of approval passes around, and the gateway opens for our journey onwards. Easing into their day handlers move on, green plastic bags daintily held by outstretched hands.

It's our first day in obedience class and Scout and I are loitering by the entrance to the field; he's exploring the scents around the gate while I hope I have the right field. We're waiting for our instructor, a woman who loves dogs and does not suffer fools, especially handlers. No one else is here. We're an hour early.

The handlers and dogs on the training programme have left for the hills and woodlands, leaving the village to slip back into its slumber. It's the place you'd want to move to: affluent, well kept. A stream babbles down the centre, tiny bridges cross it, a pub with hanging baskets. It's a long way from city life.

Scout has been studying the field through the bottom rail of the gate, his head darting left and right. I see small brown lumps bouncing along the grass – rabbits – new to Scout and an opportunity to introduce him to wildlife. We wander around the field, keeping the lead short, soft words of encouragement flowing down, small morsels of cocktail sausage offered as reward. His legs are so short his fat pink belly skims the grass. He keeps his eyes on mine and maintains a steady pace. We reach the end of the field, the rabbits now gone, Scout sniffing the ground. On our return a puppy appears out of the village hall, a tight lead pulling the Third Man. He's dressed head to toe in dazzlingly bright orange, heavy winter mountain boots, his face one huge smile of excitement and happiness. Scout and I stand enthralled by the vision, and the smile beaming out.

Others arrive and we exchange puppy names, puppy ages, puppy gender, puppy parentage. Dogs have travelled from all over England to spend three days training. No one asks any questions of the human at the other end of the lead. The Third Man instantly becomes the target for a stream of observations on his sartorial elegance and slips effortlessly into the pack.

Two handlers stand away, watching the growing mayhem of puppies trailing leads through human legs, and the rising waves of yelping as the giant knot gets tighter. They move away, calming their dogs with soft words and strokes of comfort. Today, after months of practice, they will be assessed on obedience. If they pass, they will take the field stock test, and if successful, join the training programme. In three years, they could be saving lives.

It's a big day.

The mood of the group becomes serious. Dogs brought to heel, frantic requests whispered for behaviour to be significantly modified; tension rises as nerves leach out along the line. Dogs become unsettled, sensing the handlers' nerves flowing down the lead into their psyche. Scout moves in closer to me, both of us at a loss to know what is happening.

A retriever lunges towards the end of the line and for the first time I notice the instructor, standing still, watching. The dog gets pulled back but lunges again, pulling the lead taut, the handler jerking forwards, the dog's tongue hanging and paws clawing up sods of grass, words from the handler increasingly ineffective the more desperate the scene becomes. We all step back to give a clear path.

'Down.'

The retriever drops instantly, its tail a blur of compliance, eyes blazing brightly at the instructor who calmly gives the dog a treat, says sweet words, strokes an ear, the dog rolling over in rapture.

'Some work still to do.'

The handler, ex-army, whispers 'Yes,' his eyes pleading forgiveness. All leads have shortened.

In the field we place traffic cones, hurdles, a see-saw, a long yellow tunnel. Now tied up, the dogs keep their eyes on their own handler as we gather in a circle, jostling for position. I make myself stay in line, in the middle of the circumference, and tick off character profiles: the joker, the statesman, the pro. We're all trying to have square shoulders and straight backs, the very image of strength and dependability, notwithstanding the cute puppy now chewing its leash and the odd paunch creeping over the waistband. The only female stands calmly waiting, relaxed. I mark her down as competent and hard. And what am I?

We spend the morning getting Scout walking to heel, sitting on command and working on recall, keeping distances short so we don't strain his tender limbs and joints, the closeness helping cement our bond. Training is by encouragement and reward for both dog and handler; threat is never used. For every dog and hopefully handler, this process must be fun, and the rewards firmly associated with the desired behaviour. This imprinting is the foundation of the 'find sequence' which we will eventually use to help people in distress. Each time Scout gets something right he gets a morsel as a reward. By late morning he's beginning to get the hang of the game. He's worked out the food is kept in the chalk bag on my belt. When he performs a task correctly and gets praise, his eyes flick from mine to the bag of treats.

At midday we rest; the mental energy training requires is exhausting for both of us. Scout has a small meal before being put to bed, sleep coming seconds after his body has snuggled into its soft nest. I join the others, chat about training, call-outs, the usual conversations of any like-minded group. It's very relaxing and I feel myself beginning to be more at ease.

In the afternoon we continue while the more advanced dogs work out on the equipment. There is a mix of proficiency of handler and dog in the group. Some are within a month or two of taking the obedience test, some are grappling with the down stay for ten minutes – a conundrum for the dogs: should I stay or go and find the handler? Some dogs have not found the switch for work mode, spending their time wandering away to sleep off dinner. The two dogs hoping for assessment have spent the morning being closely watched and now are gone.

More dogs arrive overnight after handlers finish their working week. There is a mix of breeds, with the most suitable dog for the work often a heated debate. No one has turned up with a poodle or a chihuahua yet, but we all live in hope. The supreme champion is the Border collie bred from working stock. The breed is a relative newcomer. Old Hemp, a tricolour bred in the Northumberland border country in the 1890s, is the ancestor of all pure-bred Border collies like Scout. He was known for his quiet work ethic and ability to control stock. The breed is generally accepted as being the most intelligent of all dogs. Inhospitable terrain and weather are no obstacle for Border collies. Their ability to work consistently in difficult conditions and over prolonged periods of time, along with their ability to think through situations, has made the breed the pre-eminent dog in search and rescue.

Scout and I make good progress during the second day. He now knows his name when I say it and is very fixed on me. I'm more relaxed. Now I know what I am doing, what is expected of me.

On the final day, there is a meeting before everyone leaves for a few more hours of training, then the drive home. The two dogs under assessment have passed both the obedience test and the field stock test and join the search dog training programme. The handlers are presented with a hi-vis dog coat and a small lime-green dog tag, both emblazoned with the words *Trainee Mountain Rescue Search Dog*. People cheer and clap. The handlers, now one half of a trainee dog team, shift from foot to foot, their eyes fixed on those embossed words, fingers absorbing their meaning.

Scout is cute, drawing attention wherever we go. Those beautiful markings, a perfectly proportioned tiny body, his loving nature. Place him on some wheels and a child could happily pull him along. Each day brings new people to meet. He follows the conversation, his eyes tracking whoever is talking, his attention total – and he loves attention. He is magnetic. It's a useful skill to have for his first official team appearance.

Each year mountain rescue teams around the country must raise money to run their operation. It pays for kit. The equipment used is highly specialised and expensive to purchase and maintain. There are the vehicles – the Land Rovers, pickups, control vans – some teams have more than half a dozen. Stretchers, ropes, helmets, jackets, medical supplies, fuel – all must be sourced and paid for. A base from which to operate, store equipment, run training. As technology develops, items need upgrading, radios go from analogue to digital, computers need up-to-date systems. It's an expensive pastime.

Many people assume mountain rescue is funded by the government. This is not the case. Teams receive no support from the government, and many argue mountain rescue is the better for it. This independence comes at a cost though: volunteers have to constantly battle to raise funds to keep helping people in distress, each team having to annually raise up to £100,000, sometimes more.

Collection tins anywhere people gather are a source of funds, as are donations from fell runners, mountain bikers, climbers and walkers, both as individuals and clubs. It's a way of paying back and being responsible in making sure support is there when needed. It is this independence and self-reliance – everyone mucking in – that forms the DNA of mountain rescue. There are other sources of funds; companies and other charitable organisations all help, particularly with the big-ticket items. You can't just walk out of a showroom with a custom-built Land Rover, it's going to cost an arm and a leg.

The most visible and most enjoyable part of fundraising for team members and supporters is the bucket rattle. This is where Scout is going to help, spending the day at Sheffield train station, looking ridiculously cute and greeting travellers.

We are there by 6.30 a.m. to catch the morning rush. Walking on to the concourse, it's big and loud. People buying coffee and tickets, checking train times, meeting travellers, trains arriving and leaving, the heavenly voice booming down. I have Scout on a short lead to keep him clear of all those feet. His head swivels as he takes in the strange environment. We have only walked a few metres across the shiny floor when Scout attracts attention; people spin around and point out the gorgeous little puppy with the big red collar and bright, confident air. By the time we reach the rest of the team we have a small following trailing us.

Scout has a long day being stroked, kissed, petted, cuddled, photographed, kissed again. Businesspeople lie on the floor in fine clothes just to grab a selfie; even the British Transport Police join in. The team announce his presence on social media which brings people on special journeys to see him, visiting during breaks from work, some several times in the day. There are a lot of young women turning up just to spend time with him. Queues form; those waiting watch Scout's latest fan tickle his tummy, sounds of pleasure blocking out station announcements. Phones are passed around for the photo op, instructions given about the best profile, waiting for Scout to perform his latest iteration in cuteness, sticking his little pink tongue out. Social media brings more donations to be dropped into the buckets, a squeaky toy, more glamour shots. At the end of the day people are travelling home and deliriously happy to see Scout still at the station, emptying their pockets and purses of spare change. It makes a huge difference to the team, thousands of pounds donated from the good people who fell in love with Scout.

As we turn into Scout's first summer, we've attended a few weekend training camps and have got ourselves into a nice routine. He loves the weekends away, all the people, the games we play, the conveyor belt of treats for doing well. Camp is usually a bunkhouse, some grander than others. The dogs sleep in cars and vans, handlers clucking around them at bedtime tucking them in with a bedtime story. I spend the run up to the weekends preparing our food, hill kit and sleeping gear. Being married to a vegetarian means when we are away, we indulge in steak and bacon.

I rise early at camp, easing slowly into the day. The older handlers are about, grunting good morning, minds working through the hours ahead. After breakfast, I walk with Scout. We chat about training, the things we did well yesterday. He has his breakfast while I pack my rucksack with food, water, dog bowl, and chat to handlers and dogsbodies. There's a briefing session – who goes where. People leave in convoy, those new clinging to the vehicle in front desperate not to be left behind.

In the evening, I talk to other handlers about our day, ask a few questions and sift through the advice I need and what I think I don't. I make notes of reflection, writing down weather conditions, who was present, what went well or what needs attention. These habits leave me free to concentrate on Scout. At bedtime, he gets a juicy carrot and I tell him how much he is loved. For me, bed by 9 p.m. with a chocolate Hobnob, or maybe two.

With days lengthening, Scout's limbs grow, and his body knits together. Longer walks raise the activity levels and lead to an increase in food. We hit the local pet store where Scout finds treasure in the sweepings underneath the bottom treat shelf, his time spent headfirst in the tight gap, his backside and legs sticking out and a tail happily polishing the floor.

Exercising Scout is something I am careful with. Border collies are prone to hip displacement, where the joints and surrounding tissue structures have not been allowed to grow slowly enough and consequently fail. The vet stipulates a walk of five minutes for every month of age. We take it easy; Scout will be eighteen months old before we take on a full day walk.

At home he pushes his explorations further afield. He's finally worked out the staircase. While still a little tentative, his growing body has given him the confidence to go up and down, opening the whole house to him and, with four floors and three flights of stairs, it's good hill repetition work. He's sleeping less and has more energy that we burn off with frequent walks around the streets and obedience work in the garden.

My usual mountain rescue team training continues. I begin brushing up my core skills for assessment later in the year, the team having added, removed or refined some of the requirements, adding another night of training. I need to make time for Alison, Monty, Olly and myself. We get out for a short walk on Sundays, taking the Trangia to cook breakfast, relax watching the clouds go by and talk over our days. Call-outs keep at a steady level:

people lost, mountain bikers crashing, injured walkers, the odd climber hitting the deck. With a major forest mountain bike track in our area, weekends are busy. Quick extraction to hospital is key. Feedback from A&E shows that many casualties have life-threatening internal injuries, the result of feeling wind rushing through the hair and trees flashing past, and at the last minute seeing the huge tree or boulder refusing to step aside.

The longest line of blackened gritstone on our patch is Wharncliffe Crags, overlooking a wide boulder field. While some teams close by will attend a crag rescue several times a week, for my team it is a sporadic event. The last crag rescue was in a storm – thunder, lightning and lashing rain making for an atmospheric rescue of a climber who had plummeted feet first down the crag face, their lower limbs splintering into shards. To add a little spice amidst the storm passing overhead, the safest way out was not across the boulder field, but along the top of the crag, below twitching powerlines.

Becoming a dog handler more than doubles this commitment. Search dogs and handlers, while part of a team, are also a national asset and can be deployed anywhere in the country, making them unique in the mountain search and rescue community.

Scout has had a growth spurt and we have run out of garden. We move to a large, grassed area in Hillsborough Park where twice each day we practise our routine of heel walks, down stay and recall. The park is full of distractions – dogs and people, lots of picnics, and children running around screaming and having a good time. I notice no one is using the tennis courts in the morning. The cage would be perfect for our work, the area large enough to do everything we need, so I begin using them and it works well. Being away from the bustle gives us a calm space and helps us both focus on the down stay without fear that Scout may wander away.

Our days run on tramlines. It's gentle and immersive; the more time we spend together the stronger our bond is forged.

'Turn.'

This is new. We didn't expect to be doing turns today. Heel walking is going well, we are both relaxed, having fun. There is a hedge looming toward us, and we've been told to turn rather than stop. I wheel us around, not quite dragging Scout, but there is little elegance in the manoeuvre. We make it round, walking triumphantly back to the instructor while other handlers look on appreciatively. We stop. Scout sits and I give him a small piece of sausage.

'Is that it?'

I've no idea what I have done wrong.

'A bit of sausage. And that's it?' The final three words punched out leaving bruised holes in the air. Handlers fold their arms and settle back.

'How much time do you spend with Scout?' Scout, on hearing his name moves toward the instructor and is immediately commanded to sit. He sits instantly. A hand jabs me.

'Treat.'

I fumble.

'Treat.' This time with an edge.

I place a small piece of cocktail sausage in the hand. It looks small, cheap and pathetic. Scout snaffles it up as the air is suddenly filled with a high-pitched trill.

'Good boy.'

Scout slips into adoration mode, loving this new experience.

'Treat.'

I'm feeding the demanding hand as fast as I can while the titters from the other handlers begin rolling across the field that has become exceedingly small.

'Why are you rewarding Scout with cheap tasteless sausage? That's the best he deserves, is it?'

The instructor now has Scout's full attention.

'I thought … '

'Thought! He needs praise, needs to know you are pleased. This is supposed to be rewarding.'

I'm not sure what to say, so stand rooted to the spot. The others grin. Another poke in the ribs snaps me back into the torture area.

'And put some life in your voice and movement. It's like watching an undertaker. You're not one of them, are you?'

'One of what?'

'An undertaker, for crying out loud.' Laughter booms across the field. I shake my head.

'Watch me.' The instructor takes the lead, Scout trots happily at the side, neither in front nor behind, enjoying all the attention. I watch, trying not to look like an undertaker. The instructor looks back.

'Well, come on. You won't learn back there.' The other handlers wave me on with little flicks of their hand, faces red with merriment.

Scout is loving it. The twitter of words, the constant feed from the sausage machine holding him in place. His only purpose and desire is to comply with the instructor's command, the control plain to see. At the hedge they wheel round in a perfectly executed arc and smoothly return ending with a perfect sit. Everything simply perfect. I glance over at the others, heads shaking slowly.

'Loose lead.'

We hear those words many times in obedience class. A tight lead says poor control, the dog taking the handler for a walk. And perhaps, a commentary on the handler's approach to life. A person who has a loose lead on life is relaxed, content, in control of what matters. It sounds a little new age, but all that gentleness passes down the lead to a calm, confident dog.

I try to create a calm environment at home, no upheavals, no sudden sounds. The more I work at this the more the atmosphere becomes tense and forced, especially for Alison. She sits me down and explains how home feels. 'Unfriendly,' is the word she slowly, gently releases from her lips. 'You're losing sight of what is important,' she says, 'our happiness, all of us, the dogs' too, and yours.'

I try to make sense of what is happening, talk it through with some friends. One points out how angry I seem at the world. How unapproachable my face is, what she calls a 'fuck-off face'. I talk about what is happening in my life, how tense things have become, what I am trying to achieve, but at what cost to me and my loved ones at home? I take a well-worn path around the subject until, with nowhere else to go, I finally arrive at what is disturbing me. She listens in silence and watches me. She tells me some of her day, the recent past. We pass back and forth for a while. Finally, she says my troubles aren't the world's fault, or Alison's. 'Get some professional help,' she says, 'because what you are doing isn't sustainable.' It might even mean giving up Scout.

Team members drag themselves out of bed in the darkness of a winter night, peering into the blackness that hammers sleet against the windows. They set foot on a storm-ravaged hill to look for someone they do not know and will probably never meet. This is not the behaviour of normal people.

Well-being is an issue in mountain rescue. The need to be seen, to be in control, coping, is a powerful mask. Layering that with trauma, harsh conditions, and mixing in the daily life of family and work – it's a lot to take on. Help in many forms is there: a chat over a pint, a curry with a few mates, dark humour after a trying call-out, a day on the hill, the love of those closest. Sometimes professional help is needed, and sometimes that need is ignored.

It takes me time to find help, to begin unpicking a life. Slowly, unknowingly, the search for me begins. I'm reminded to wear life like a loose jacket, and I think about the loose lead. I'm closer to a solution than I realise, a thread that I have teased for years, and like any journey off the map the way forward will come unexpectedly.

As summer eases into autumn, Scout and I have established a smooth routine. Twice a day we walk the neighbourhood, lead loose, enter the park, lead off. Scout walks to heel as I keep up a stream of encouragement and reward. We practise the 'sit' command, the recall, and repeat and repeat to imprint the habits. Obedience builds empirically, so we don't move on until we have solidified what is behind us. The most difficult command to master is the 'down stay for ten minutes'. It causes the most stress in handlers and consequently the dog. Many a handler has tensely waited, and prayed, for the ten minutes to be over, only to find at the end that the dog is nowhere to be seen.

The tennis courts are full, so we decamp to the large sports field. Around the edge are trees and low hedges that are perfect for watching Scout in position. It's still warm, the field full of young families picnicking, children running free, dogs chasing balls. Lots of distraction and noise. I figure if we can do it here the assessment will be a walk in the park.

Scout is all long limbs and sharp corners, and huge ears like sound mirrors. Road walking has thickened and blackened the soles of his pads. I'm getting to know his idiosyncrasies, paying closer attention to how he responds to my voice. Soft, calm and gentle has a significantly greater positive effect.

A big step has been changing the reward to roasted liver. Scout loves it, though it's created a major issue in our vegetarian home. Alison is disgusted. In fairness, she has a point. The house is like a tannery. I am exiled to a spot on Loxley Common, cooking in a charcoal barbecue tray. The smoke gives the liver even more pungency, enticing the Common's dogs, their red-faced owners breaking out of bushes, trousers ripped, hands bloodied. I offer a convoluted explanation, aware it's completely mad. In the end, I cook at night, producing batches that last two weeks. Local wildlife is my only company; the local youth give me a wide berth. I chop the liver into a plastic box then clear away the bottles of cider and silver nox canisters the kids have left. Then home and a shower.

The down stay progresses well. I begin by laying him down, facing me, head up, remaining like this for a minute to settle. Then I back away, repeating 'stay'. Then I go back and reward with lots of liver and some high-pitched praise that draws attention we ignore. We keep doing this until I can stand fifty metres away from his prone body. Once we have that cemented, I begin scribing a widening arc left and right, eventually drawing a full circle around him. Over weeks we hone this until we can confidently do it for more than ten minutes, even with children playing nearby and the odd dog coming up to Scout for a natter.

The next step is to build the out-of-sight imprint. I move away from Scout after five minutes of him staying down. Gradually. A few seconds then a minute at a time. Sometimes Scout's face appears around the tree I'm hiding behind, so we reset and go again. Every time it goes right, he gets a reward and praise. We get beyond ten minutes – we only need five, but I want to be doubly sure.

At half-term, the park is full of mums and dads with their children playing ball games, eating ice cream, having a happy time. Hiding behind a bush to watch Scout doesn't seem like a good idea. I stick to a tree, nonchalantly leaning against it out of sight of Scout, who is a hundred metres away in the middle of the field. The park attendant asks what I'm doing.

'Training my dog.'

'What dog?'

'The one sat in the middle of the field. I hope.'

'Hiding behind a tree by the ice cream van.'

'I'm just trying to train my dog for mountain work.'

'In a park! You need to find somewhere else.'

My watch says it's been seventeen minutes since I left Scout. Sticking my head around the tree, he's still there – head, ears, eyes alert. I whistle him over and he bounds across the grass to a huge hug, squeals of praise and a handful of liver. We leave. But not before Scout gets a large Mr. Whippy.

At the next weekend camp, I ask if we can take the test; the other two local dogs have already passed obedience. We're told no. We're not ready. So, we continue.

. . .

I'm confident I have control of Scout and can work on the field stock test. The major hurdle is getting him near enough to sheep to train him without him chasing or harming them. I can't just walk into a field of sheep and let him loose, farmers have a thing about that.

Happily, the Yorkshire Sculpture Park is nearby. Lots of free-roaming sheep, people, dogs; the grounds full of art, Henry Moore and Barbara Hepworth. Andy Goldsworthy's *Shadow Stone Fold* – a large sheepfold installation – is perfect for us. It forms a solid barrier between the sheep and Scout, so he can get used to their presence and I can work out how to train him. The flock looks content around people and dogs, so I reason they are far less likely to be jumpy and run.

Each day we sit in the sheepfold chatting, playing ball, going through basic obedience, keeping Scout's mind focused while the sheep watch trying to work out what this odd pair are doing. If he looks at the sheep, I tell him 'no' in a soft, calm voice, stretching out the 'n' and 'o' into a non-threatening drawl. He flashes me a look. We settle for a few minutes, me stroking his coat and limbs while chatting about what I see, other than sheep.

After a few days of watching the sheep watching us we are relaxed enough to take a lead walk across the edge of the flock, fifty metres or more between us. The sheep remain, watching closely. Scout begins to huff and puff, cheeks blowing out, hackles raised. The sheep remain firm but wary. I give him the command 'no' and pull him back, but he's crossed some line and immediately sends more bad vibes to the flock, whose front line stomp the ground in warning. They hold us in their gaze, throwing a gauntlet that immature Scout cannot resist. The lead goes tighter and tighter as he strains toward them; a guttural foaming grinds out of his mouth as he lunges. I shout a sharp 'NO'. Everything goes still and heavy. People have stopped to look. A black masse of crows rise from oaks to circle, calling out 'murder, murder'. The sheep have scattered. They regroup under a large beech by the old churchyard. Scout has returned to heel and now lies in submission. Crouching, I smooth his brow.

We take a walk around a lake to decompress. When we return the sheep have drifted down from the church. As Scout begins paying attention, I release the ultimate deterrent. 'No' brings him back in line. We call it a day and head home.

The following week we walk slowly past the flock, the 'no' getting softer and earlier as I learn to read Scout's body language, and he understands the new command. By the end of the week, it's sufficient to just clear my throat.

It's still warm when we set our base under the beech by the churchyard. Against the tree, Scout by my side, we enjoy the peace of the landscape, relaxing in the bright sunshine admiring the colours of the autumn leaf and the dappled light playing around us. Scout watches birds flit to and fro, snoozes a little. The sheep graze quietly down the hill. Scout rests chin on paws, no anxiety. Sheep, dog and handler placidly let time flow by.

I tell him to stay and walk away. He maintains position, eyes on me. The sheep show so little concern, I'm sure it's because they know we don't pose a threat. I move slowly, taking my time to stroll back to Scout and pick up his lead, then turn and walk him through the flock keeping my pace even and Scout close but the lead loose. If he looks at the sheep I softly say 'no', stretching it out until it is lost in the warm breeze. A few sheep give us space, some stand their ground, none run. It's all very sedate and gentle. I'm quiet. The ultimate deterrent stays in its box.

The greatest danger for a sheep chase is the lone sheep. Hidden in bracken or behind a rock, enjoying a moment of solitude, being confronted by a dog without warning. Both springing up in alarm, the sheep taking flight and the dog, after regaining its composure, thinking *game on*. A search dog must resist this impulse, ignore the adrenaline coursing through its body, ignore the animal in flight. Sheep, hares, birds, deer, cattle, all must be treated the same by Scout.

Come September we get the chance to test Scout with the other two local dogs at a farm. A dozen sheep are held in a sheepfold; high drystone walls prevent them jumping out. Watching are handlers, dogsbodies, the farmer and his dogs. I lead Scout into the fold and slip his lead off. He looks at me, then the sheep huddled together in a corner, eyes fixed on their old foe. 'Stay,' I command, then step out. The sheep watch Scout. Scout looks at me. The flock begins rotating around the walls, Scout in the centre of the washing machine looking very confused. I call him. Glad to be out of it he runs through the sheep to my feet. Then his toy is placed in a corner and the sheep pressed over it, he dives in on command and comes out with the toy, the sheep scattering like snooker balls. We've completed the test and no sheep have been harmed. We stand around watching the other two dogs, letting the tension ease out. All three dogs pass. While I am delighted, something gnaws away.

That night I get a call from the Second Man. We discuss the day. He's more experienced than me having trained a dog before; he suggests the test was not to the standard. That's the gnawing something. *The standard.* I've allowed myself to be swept along on a tide of haste and desire. I've equated training with passing a test, rather than meeting the standard. Neither of us can let the pass stand. The Third Man has been put forward for two tests now, passing both, but not at the standard. Understandably, he isn't happy at taking another.

At the Chew Valley training camp in October, we go through another test, this time in a large inbye pasture where there is plenty of room for the large flock to move. Scout attains the standard, but we still await formal assessment.

At eight months old, Scout is firming up in all directions. Another year or so and all the bones, tendons, sinew and muscle will have knitted together. He can now walk for forty minutes giving us freedom from the local park. We have Loxley Common nearby, part of a hunting ground centuries back, then caught in the Industrial Revolution, now returning to a wilder landscape of heath, woodland and quarries. It's popular with dog walkers, horse riders, bird watchers and couples looking for a little privacy. There's an abundance of wildlife: foxes, badgers, rabbits, deer and birds. We take our morning walks there, Scout runs free through the woodland and coppices. He's becoming popular with the other dog walkers, but other dogs – non-working dogs – he ignores.

November brings cooler temperatures and dark nights. Every year mountain rescue pumps out a message for walkers to be prepared with torches, maps, food, drink, the right clothing, and every year the teams are called from their beds to help someone to safety. People don't intend to be rescued. Teams have a generally pragmatic view of call-outs, the plus being some wonderful night-time wanders. Technology helps with many of the incidents. Smartphones can be used to pinpoint a casualty and, if they are in a fit state, they can be talked off a hill without the team member getting out of bed. There will always be instances where phones cannot help and the old technology – a dog and a grumpy handler – come into their own.

We make our way to Brecon for a training weekend, a landscape that is like the moorland and crag of the Peak District, only bigger, rounder and steeper. I'm hoping this might be the camp we move on to the training programme, though no one has said anything. It's an assessment weekend, dogs and handlers looking to get on to the call-out list after three years of work. There is tension; handlers stand nervously around waiting to be sent to an assessment area.

As dog teams are being assessed for the call-out list this weekend, manpower is stretched. The dogs in obedience join those in stage one of the training programme. Around us are the assessment areas, a dominating and – for some handlers – terrifying landscape. Occasionally a handler will abandon their operational assessment here, unable to deal with the difficult terrain and terror in their mind. I witnessed this happen in 2015, three years of work thrown away in one moment of overwhelming trauma. One day, we will work this area, perhaps in assessment or even a call-out. For now, we are on a flat moor by a lay-by with a butty wagon doing a brisk trade in bacon sandwiches.

People run off on to the moor screaming, jumping up from dugouts, waving arms, shouting a dog's name. Dogs shoot from handlers, racing across the moor to an explosion of movement and noise as they find a human and get a reward. If we ever pass obedience, this will be our next step.

Scout is getting excited by all the activity, so I play with him, grinding away at heel work, recall and down stay. The instructor leading the stage one dogs comes over. He's no nonsense, to the point of not suffering fools. He wants to know how it's going. I tell him we're really good, commanding Scout to drop down. He does; my stomach knot loosens.

'We're ready for our test.' I say this as a fact. I'm a long way outside my comfort zone.

'Let's see then.'

'What, now?'

'Said you were ready. Let's see. Over there: walk to heel, lead on.'

I snatch the opportunity. Off we walk, Scout doing a lovely walk to heel, lead loose. With all the noise coming from the barking dogs and squealing dogsbodies, and lorries crawling up the long road out of the valley with gears crunching and engines straining to a scream, I'm impressed he is so completely at ease. Handlers begin to watch. I try to relax.

'Now take the lead off and walk back to heel, towards me.'

We do, perfectly. I might even have a smile.

'Tell him to sit and you walk to me.'

I do. Scout sits, his eyes on me as I walk to the instructor, forcing my head not to look back. When I reach the instructor and turn, Scout is still in position, eyes fixed on me. I almost squeal.

'Call him to you.'

I do. Scout bounds across the moor, the tufts of grass too high for his little legs so he slaloms his way to heel.

'Leave him there and come with me.'

I do. Scout plants himself down, back straight, feet firmly in front. We walk, a long way. I glance back to see if he is still there. He is. My confidence rises.

'Why are you looking back?'

'To make sure he has not moved.' I know this is the wrong answer and wait for the recoil.

'You said you were ready.'

'Yes, we are.' I feel the opportunity slipping.

'Well, leave him be. Call him and, when I say, put him in the down stay position.'

I turn, call Scout. He's charging towards me, everyone is watching, he's too fast, my heart is racing, I fight the urge to put him down.

'Now.'

'Down.' Scout hits the ground, body straight, paws forward, eyes boring into mine.

'Leave him there for five minutes.'

Scout and I remain rooted to our spots, eyes locked together, one team.

'Follow me.'

We drop into a deep hollow, where I'm to stay out of sight for five minutes. The instructor walks off. I lie back. Listen to the traffic, smell the bacon, hear the instructor telling someone they need to be quicker with the reward. The cold wind cuts into me, pushing me further into my belay jacket. I can't believe this is happening.

Colour catches my eye on the other side of the valley; a line of people in jeans, trainers and fashion tops make their way up the slabs to the summit of Pen y Fan. The sky looks like it's just holding on to the rain. I wonder how many call-outs there are on this route. Close to the road, man-made paths, easy going, no gear, carrier bags. After all there's a butty wagon at the start – what could possibly go wrong?

Time has stopped, the planets stand and watch. Any minute I expect Scout's face to appear at the rim of the hole asking me what I think I am doing. It's the instructor I see first; my heart sinks.

'Call your dog.'

Scrambling out of the hollow, Scout is still in position his eyes glued to the spot he last saw me. I'm so overjoyed when I scream his name. He comes full speed and jumps into my arms for a hug as tight as can be and way too many kisses.

'That's it. You've passed obedience, well done.'

'Is that it?'

'Yes. You're mine now.'

Over at the line of stage one handlers we get pats and congratulations. I don't have any words, just smiles, loving Scout, plying him with treats, reliving the triumph. When we get back to base the obedience instructor comes over to congratulate us.

'You knew?'

'I thought you were both ready and you didn't let me down.'

I've been saving a can of sardines for a special occasion; Scout has never tasted them, so he pays close attention to his evening meal. As he eats, I stroke his back and tell him how proud I am.

The narrow lanes wind along the bottom of the valley and the van I'm trying to tail keeps whipping out of sight. The roads are damp and slick with leaf fall; flashes of pasture and buildings pulse through gaps. I have no idea where we are or where we are going but it doesn't matter. After yesterday I'm in high spirits.

There's a hill farm, tucked tightly into a small cleft. A track leads from the bright white farmhouse, beyond a row of neat cottages, to disappear through a gate on to rising green fields fringed with autumnal oak and hawthorn. Gold and red leaf drip with last night's Welsh rain; the sun shines brightly from a clear blue sky that feeds a chill into the air. It is quiet; only chattering birds and the babble of soft water tumbling over rocks. It's beautiful.

As we walk up the field, packs on backs, dogs on leads, we chat about how it's going, what has worked well and what hasn't, what trials we have overcome. I have a feeling that we're all straining to get ahead; no one feels they are not ready. It's a big group, dogs from all over the country, as much a mix as the handlers, the different tongues turning this corner of a Welsh valley into Babel.

Rising higher, the group bunches up. People walk into the backs of others like shunting trains, dogs become tangled. There, in the centre of the ridge is a large flock of sheep, who, spotting the dogs, turn and stare, hard. We stare back, fidgeting and murmuring, gesticulating at the sheep.

Our base – known forever as 'the Office' no matter where in the country we are – is beneath an old blackthorn. Sorting out gear we're told to get ready for a field stock test; there is to be no training. We stare blankly at the speaker. No one has said anything about a test. No one is prepared, despite what we were saying on the walk up.

Scout sits by my pack, his nose pecking at the smell coming off the ridge. The flock is moved into position down the spine of the field. Silence has descended. I kneel and stroke Scout whispering sweet nothings into his ears. His nose twitches, nostrils flaring as he takes in the scent-laden air. I've never seen him do that before. I study closely. He keeps his nose moist with his tongue, glistening with tiny bubbles of saliva.

A shout. A dog has slipped its lead and is bounding towards the sheep who are now scattering from the ridge and throwing themselves over the nearest wall into the next field, lots of bleating and stone clattering, a stream of obscenities coming from the handler in hot pursuit; the dog ignores pleas, the lead bouncing wildly in excitement. The circus moves out of view, the sound of their continued presence ricocheting through the valley. We watch in silence. 'There but for the grace go ourselves', and our future as a search dog team. Despondency seeps through the group. Tense glances, raised eyebrows, check and recheck of dog's lead and anchor. No one speaks.

The sheep are brought back; the errant dog and its handler make their apologies and leave. We won't see them again. The day no longer looks bright and beautiful.

We are the first to be tested. It isn't what I wanted, it isn't what any of us want. I can feel the tension drain out of the others. They wish me luck, tell me to stay calm. I return a weak smile, feel the knot in my stomach, and my legs disconnect from my brain.

Recall is first. Scout on one side of the flock and me on the other. The instructor takes Scout and I make the long trek around the perimeter of the field, so I don't disturb the flock, my legs folding with each step. Scout watches until I am out of sight. Between us a large creamy mound watches both of us. The sheep are hemmed in by the other handlers and bristle with agitation. The wind has dropped. The colours are green, cream and blue. At the signal I call Scout. He appears, heading up the field towards the ridge, his body pointing to where my voice came from. The clear ground between him and the sheep disappears fast; the sheep stomp a warning, still he comes. His body filling my frame, my whole being pulls at the thread that holds us together. He hits the ridge and the sheep scatter like a smashed atom. He keeps coming, sees me, picks up speed – all around, creamy mounds streak across the grass filling the hills with tortured braying. Scout clears the ridge, the sheep behind him now, and rushes into my arms knocking me over as I launch his ball toy and squeal with delight.

I lean back against the wall and cuddle Scout. The day is bright again.

We throw a ball into the middle of the flock, Scout's eyes growing wider as he follows the trajectory. Let it settle, then release Scout. He charges into the flock, too fast for most of them to move before he is lost in the middle. When they have cleared enough space, I see Scout nosing the ground for his toy; I lose him in the maelstrom of wool. I cannot see. The flock slides to one side to reveal Scout lying down on the ground, his paws holding to the sky his toy, his eyes lost to his prize. The sheep regroup in a corner and glare at Scout throwing his toy around. I give him some liver, tell him how good he is. He checks my hand for more, then the grass. Satisfied he goes back to his toy.

I settle back against the wall again, drained.

One last test. I leave Scout in a down stay on the ridge and walk to the edge of the field with his toy. The sheep are corralled by the other handlers and moved towards Scout. He looks at me, then the sheep, then me. 'Stay,' I mutter to myself. 'Stay.' As the gap between him and the sheep closes the handlers pick up the pace until a shout signals the charge and the sheep are driven on to Scout. The flock falters and stumbles as it splits to get around him; I lose sight of him in all the wool and hooves. Then I see his face, his eyes huge and distended, but he waits, then I lose him again. When the stampede is over, I see him lying in the same place. Bits of turf and soil cover his body; his eyes are rigidly fixed on me. When I call, he launches out with relief vibrating through his body.

I lie on the ground for him to pounce, his paws pounding my body, his nose digging for his toy.

Handlers raise their hands in approval at Scout's performance. I cannot be any prouder of him, how perfect he has been all weekend. Overcome with emotion I wipe a few tears, hear the instructor telling me we have passed the field stock test.

The remaining hours of that day I rest with Scout beneath the trees, reflecting on our journey. The farm where he was born, that first training camp, the hours in the park, all of it meaningful. I watch the other dogs, help herd sheep. It's the happiest I have been in a long time. That evening Scout gets more sardines, and more kisses, and we sleep and sleep.

Sunday morning, we gather for the briefing. They announce who has passed the test and registered on to the training programme. Scout and I get a mention and the reward of a small green dog tag, and a bright green hi-vis dog coat, both bearing the legend *Trainee Mountain Rescue Search Dog*.

The words feel good.

· · ·

Humans are programmed to seek sanctuary. Survival takes hold, we make decisions based on preserving life. It's what search and rescue relies on, humans acting as programmed.

The time between safe and unsafe is a thought, and no thought. The shift happens in a step, a hand hold, the seconds between dusk and nightfall, attention drifting from the vital turn, the hubris of ignorance, the inept, the unlucky, the fearful. The human.

Step across a rivulet, the black water fringed with a web of silver threads, snow draping tiny banks, the water narrow enough to place a foot across without breaking stride. How pretty winter looks, even in its anger – the last memory before cold and darkness envelop the brain then snap it back into the world with a whiplash of light. The first thought: why is snow red?

Lost walkers are pulled by ghosts along a contour-easing passage – a sheep trod, the easy route. Cold, hungry, lost. Comforting technology pulled away as the last bar blinks out, no signal no matter how high the stretch. Keep on moving, fatal.

A lost child has sense beyond the ego of grown men and women. Tiredness means shelter sought. A bush, an overhanging rock, an old barn, a pile of soft leaf, anywhere they can rest and make ready for daylight. You hope.

A lost soul. A tree chosen months before. A quiet woodland dell full of beauty and peace. A bough strong enough to hold eternity. The peace of the day, family around the table, unknowing until morning. The world falling silent.

Broken limbs, the peat bog, the hidden hole, the fingers too tired to hold. The weightless fall, time tearing off, voices fluttering on a breeze. A loved one walking a hospital floor, past beds and other loved ones. The promise never to do it again, sell the gear, fingers and toes crossed.

And there are those that do not know they are lost. And not all are lost.

A search begins with a call to the police; someone is lost or missing. There is a distinction between the two. Missing is an unexpected absence reported by others. Lost is mostly reported by those that are, lost. It might seem a semantic, but this dictates how a call-out unfolds and the allocation of resources.

Technology has made rescue a little less of a gamble. Smartphones with a signal can be interrogated for a position and the casualty talked to safety. Being met by a group of red jackets can be comforting for those that thought they may never see civilisation again. Satellite trackers can issue alerts and pinpoint a casualty's location, without the need for a casualty to activate the call. Drones can spot the heat balloon of a human body from high above in minutes.

Lost is easier to find, as long as they don't try to extract themselves from trouble, reach for redemption. The benighted when the clocks go back, the overwhelmed by conditions, the confused by terrain, the inexperienced. All can be found. Just stay calm. Panic is the enemy leading to poor decisions and exhaustion of physical and mental resources, as the lost flail through thick vegetation, stumble over rough terrain, make a sketchy descent, chilled to the bone crossing icy water.

The missing are not lost. They have vanished, not where they were supposed to be when expected. They could be overwhelmed by conditions, injured or safe but whereabouts unknown. Establish possible locations, develop a search plan, put boots and paws on the ground. More added, like an expanding balloon as likely places are searched and nothing found, the search ever widening. The only limit is when extreme weather or danger puts rescuers' lives at risk.

The best resource a search manager has in all weathers is a search dog. A search dog team operates away from other search parties, to give the dog's nose clean uncontaminated ground. The team – dog, handler, often a navigator – can search large areas quickly and efficiently, with a high degree of certainty.

Mountain rescue has detailed behavioural profiles of missing people: children, vulnerable, experienced, inexperienced, professional, amateur, foolhardy. Combining intelligence with knowledge of local terrain and weather conditions, skilled team members are capable of moving unsupported for prolonged periods through difficult conditions at any time of day. Because of this, the search skills of mountain rescue are often called on by the police to search difficult urban areas. Not all searches are in a mountain wilderness.

When a search ends, the team stood down, members and dogs return to their homes and lives. For the families of those being sought there is joyous relief or a lifetime of questions.

The green pastures of obedience are behind us. We have stepped across the hard border of assessment, and before us, a towering yellow moor beneath a grey sky. The workplace of a search dog team.

I'm nervous and try not to show it. Impostor syndrome has kicked in and I'm sure we didn't pass and soon will be sent back to obedience class with our tails between our legs, my past conditioning scrambling for a hold. The Second Man and Third Man join me. I wonder if they feel the same. I give myself a talking to and step on to the tightrope that stretches ahead.

From now on we train with a dogsbody (body, for short) – a human acting as a casualty for dogs to find. It's the most important role in the development of a search dog team; without bodies nothing can happen. As we gather, bodies make a beeline for Scout's nose pressed against the van window. Fingers and soft words tap. I open the door and Scout plays to the gallery, the stroking hands and nuzzled noses, his head soon slick with kisses, the sweet sounds of gorgeous and beautiful please him. Each body tests the tolerance of the next in line, stretching their time with Scout beyond the norms of polite society. When Scout's fan club finally drifts away, I give him a kiss, hold him tight and feel the impostor slink back into the shadows.

A body has a strong connection with the outdoors: walkers, climbers, runners, all with a stoical resilience to foul weather and wet noses. Their role is to act as a casualty for the dog and, when found, to reward the dog with play, with treats, whatever the dog needs. It means turning adults into children – playtime really is playtime. In the early stages it involves running around a moor jumping and squealing, getting up, lying down, timing the reward exactly right – it's exhausting. The pleasantest role is with the operational dogs. A long walk up a mountain, a nice spot to lie down, relax, read a book, wait to be found, perhaps once or twice a day. Of course, in a storm it isn't like that. It's miserable.

A good body makes training easier, enjoyable, fun. Bodies are prepared for extremes, squeezing down fairy holes, hiding in dense foliage, up trees. They bring their own gear, mats, sleeping bags, old clothing, operate a radio, take instructions, offer information. A good body will note what the dog did, how it found them, any titbits that can be gold to a handler. Many come in pairs, married, partners, back year after year, becoming a major part of a dog's development from puppy to operational.

The cold wind rolling across the moor tingles my face, drawing tears down my cheeks. We are in a line with the others, each dog wearing their green hi-vis training jacket, nose twitching. The handlers stand in layers of red, the dogsbodies in tatty, drab layers to mingle with the land, hold off the cold and damp. We hold out the reward each dog works with – the display of meats, biscuits and toys – for our allocated body. Ours is a bubbly mountaineering instructor who kneels at Scout's paws catching him off guard with a high-pitched squeal that tears him away from the delights of the deli counter, his name slicing through his brain. Her face disappears behind her hands, 'peek-a-boo', the 'BOO' pinning Scout's ears back, his eyes widening, paws dancing, head swaying left and right. Good fun.

The moor rumbles as bodies tempt dogs, and dogs insist on more. Scout joins in; his first bark at a body gets him a high-pitched squeal and smothered in hugs. He copies the other dogs, barking furiously, the moor alive with confusion and movement. It's manic, amazing. I stand and laugh.

We work all morning getting Scout used to playing with these large children who run around letting go of their inhibitions at full volume. As therapy goes, this is the best it can get.

This is the footings for the foundation of the find sequence, when Scout tells me he has found a casualty and will guide me in.

First, Scout has to learn to ask for his reward, to bark when required, to 'speak'. I ask him to speak. He looks blank. I try again; he looks confused. Try something else. The body curls up tight on the ground, says 'speak'; I bark, she jumps; I get Scout's reward. Scout is perplexed. We repeat until Scout starts to bark each time I get the reward of liver and he gets nothing. He is furious that he is not in the loop, his head swivelling madly as he tracks the treats from the body into my mouth. I tell him to speak, his bark uncoils the body, nuggets of leathery liver are snaffled before the cold wind hits them.

We switch to the body commanding 'speak'. Each time Scout barks he gets a reward. The body curls into a ball, the reward held tight inside; Scout must bark; the body springs out like a jack-in-the-box – high volume, lots of movement – then Scout gets a reward. Scout soon latches on to the bark–reward system.

It's exhausting hyperactive work for the body: lots of running around, jumping, making noise, playing with the dog, all designed to make the reward high value. The dogs react differently to each body – some like manic, some gentle – the only rhyme or reason the dog's personality. No one has ever found the ceiling of a dog wanting more.

I cannot do any of this on my own at home. The experience of local handlers and bodies will be invaluable. A group train one evening a week and on Sunday mornings in the south of the Peak District. With fewer dogs we can concentrate on building the reward mechanism. Hopefully, in time, Scout will instinctively know what to do, and be fiercely insistent I listen.

Extending the space between Scout and the body, making Scout move further before he speaks, means the body has a central role and needs to be fit for the jumping around, and quick on their feet so that Scout always associates the reward with his barking. It doesn't end with a morsel of liver, there are minutes of intense play between the dog and body, increasing the pleasure for both. It's mainly the young or the super fit who fill this role. The bodies with a few more years are perfect for dogs who are further on in their careers.

Scout is becoming more independent now he speaks, a lot more talkative at home too. I think he's realised he's different to Monty and Olly, maybe even special, and he's growing in confidence. I nurture this by giving him little search tasks to find a treat when we are out, rewarding with my admittedly lowered level of hyperactivity, strengthening his skill.

At national training camp we stretch distance and time between initiation and reward. My role is to release Scout to the body and support him with encouragement. I spend my time praising, squealing delight when he speaks and standing to one side as he plays with the body. I am now Scout's bag carrier, cheerleader and treat supplier.

In most search dog areas, a local handler organises local training and acts as instructor to newer dogs. It's usually, but not always, the one who has most years on the hill and probably has trained more dogs. It is an invaluable resource, passing on knowledge, helping handlers understand and progress, ensuring new dogs are up to standard. Training a dog team is not a straight line or a competition. Often it is full of frustration, sometimes for handler and dog; two steps forward, one step back. I concentrate on getting each step right before moving on, when we are told we can.

It's nice to be part of the group and get the chance to build friendships with members from other teams. I follow advice to the letter, doing exactly as I'm told. It feels like we are on our way, even if local training does seem a little chaotic. Sometimes the advice changes week to week; it's difficult to keep track. Often the change is around the reward: food is no good, then it is. Distance is too close or too far, then it isn't. I assume this is all normal, it's just different to what we do on national training weekends. And, I notice, different from what the other dogs there are doing.

The year draws to a close and I am happy. Training is going well. The team has had another year of saving people. At home, things are good. Alison continues producing her art and lecturing at the university. I've finished my first semester at university, a creative writing degree that I have long wanted to do and am enjoying immensely. Scout is settled, and while he and Olly will never be best friends they tolerate each other. Monty has taken to giving Scout a few hard three-metre stares when he gets tired of Scout annoying him.

On Christmas Day we head out for our traditional walk, a brew and some egg banjos. We sit and talk and recharge, thankful for the peace we have.

2017

The new year finds us in Aviemore – an area used by mountain rescue teams for avalanche training. The chance of an avalanche in the Peak District is remote, but it has happened. The Cairngorms are perfect for getting the dogs used to a winter mountain environment and practising winter skills.

The handlers' first task is to create shelter for the dogs from the cold winds and piercing snow that strafes the mountain; the dogs snuggle down on insulated mats, cocooned in warm jackets. Next, 'burial graves' are dug deep enough for each body; undertaking one of the most unusual jobs in the country, they need to be comfortable for several hours below the surface. Handlers dig the graves, leaving the bodies free to stay warm and dry – a sweaty body cooling down in a snowhole is not a happy body. Some play with the dogs while waiting, others bunker down out of the wind. In the grave they will have each dog's reward, a toy or treat, along with full winter kit, several mats, thick sleeping bag, bivvy bag, a collection of hats and gloves, hot drink and food, a radio and something to while away the time between finds. There is just enough room for a dog to enter in pursuit of its reward. Once a body is settled, the tomb is sealed and left to allow the body's scent to percolate into the winter landscape.

It takes time for dogs to connect human scent to a person beneath the surface. It's a process of show, repeated until the dog understands. The handler and dog work in close proximity. This is not a wide-ranging search; the handler directs the dog to patches of snow, the dog tests for scent until it finds the spot where a human is trapped. As the dog gains experience the body is placed deeper.

The first indication a body has that the dog has located them is a tiny drizzle of snow running into the tomb, then miniature avalanches, then flashes of daylight. The first gasp of fresh air is quickly extinguished by a wet black nose thrust into the opening, hoovering great draughts of cold air, withdrawing to muffled human words outside, then thrust in again, deeper. Large clumps of the tomb cover the body; two eyes appear ringed with snow. The surprise on the dog's face on seeing human eyes looking back, the realisation the smell in the icy cave is their reward, all hell breaking loose as the dog forces its way in to the cramped space, snow falling everywhere engulfing both body and dog. The voice outside shouting praise, the body praying the whole thing does not collapse, and that soon it will all be over.

The difficulty is getting the dog out. This is high-octane happiness, a whole mountainside filled with joy, walkers and mountaineers stopping to watch the dogs dig their way in. The dogs must be coerced out with promise of treats, or their toy launched out of the new opening. Or maybe that's just dogs being smart.

We will not be training for avalanche work. While Scout has learned to speak, he does not have a return indication. Locally, along with the Third Man, we've continued with run-aways, working with bodies running away from us, screaming and squealing, making sure the dog can see its reward, before body and reward disappear from view, and the handler releases the dog to find them. Although we have progressed, at times I feel we've been stuck in a groove, repeating the same exercise over and over again. I can only follow the guidance of the local handler; I don't know enough to do otherwise. We've added a twist, called a 'pop-up'. The body, hiding unseen by Scout, springs out of the ground, wailing and screaming his name. I tell Scout the body has his treat, his eyes widen, paws claw earth, he strains forward, the body drops out of sight, I release Scout, his backside a blur as he races to the place he last saw his reward. While it's good fun, this has now become the exercise we repeat ad nauseam, and Scout's sparkle has started to diminish.

Today we have a handler from another part of the country instructing us. I'm nervous because I don't want to foul up and I'm apprehensive about what he will want us to do.

His approach is relaxed, informal, slow paced. We are just going to have fun he says. We outline our progress.

The Third Man is with us, now dressed in blue. I like him. He's relaxed and doesn't take himself too seriously. The trainer asks if our dogs have a return indication. We both shake our heads. He asks why, wrong footing us. 'The handler instructing us back home says we aren't ready,' we explain. He suggests we try. We shuffle our feet and say we don't want any upset; we'll carry on doing what we do at home.

Our base is a former army Arctic training camp, set in a forest with the aroma of Scots pine, the dappled sunlight flickering with motes of forest life. It's quiet; our boots make no sound on the soft needle floor as we move silently into the beauty and serenity of this cathedral.

With the bodies hiding behind fallen trees, hunkered down in softly carpeted hollows, we go through our normal training. After a few runs our instructor suggests a return. 'Just try it. When the dog gets to the body call the dog back, get them to speak and take you to the body. When you get there tell the body to reward the dog. You have most of the sequence anyway, so let's complete it. If it doesn't work, we can go back.' I look at the Third Man. This feels exciting, a little naughty.

Unlike trailing search dogs that rely on a scent trail from an object or piece of clothing, air-scenting search dogs rely on the human body's epidermis – the outermost skin cells – and secretions, invisible to us but highly detectable to a dog's nose, flowing across the land in ever-widening coverage.

As scent seeps outward from the human body, the cells spread out in a cone shape, the base of the cone widening as it gets further from the source. The more time scent has, and the stronger the wind and thermal conditions, the longer and wider the cone becomes. It is this scent cone that operational air-scenting dogs detect and follow to the human source.

The handler's role is to place the dog perpendicular across the wind, therefore through the cone if it is present, allowing the sensitive nose to receive the maximum amount of scent, snapping it towards the source. This is called 'the strike'.

The dog will follow the narrowing scent cone for many hundreds of metres, sometimes kilometres, irrespective of terrain, weather or obstacles, until it finds the source. Then the dog will return to the handler – indicating 'the find', usually by 'speak' (barking) – then return to the body, the handler following behind. This will be repeated by the dog, the return and indication, as many times as needed until the handler arrives at the source location. Then the dog receives its reward.

This is the return indication sequence.

. . .

We practise the 'indication' first. I ask Scout to speak; he looks at me as though I'm mad. I bark. Ears prick up, eyes widen in disbelief. He looks around, for help maybe. I bark again and say 'speak'. Scout does a little dance on the spot. I say 'speak'. Scout barks. We're both as surprised as each other. I fumble for a treat, drop it. Scout searches for the brown morsel in the brown floor, hoovers it up and looks at me. 'Speak.' Another bark, another treat. Now I can't stop him barking even when I don't have a treat ready. It has taken thirty minutes to produce his 'indication'.

The body has been told not to move until they hear me say 'reward', then follow the usual play. I know where they are; if anything goes wrong, I can guide Scout in for a successful outcome. It's the first time I have come across errorless training – the dog always gets a good result even if it must be manufactured. It's positive, simple and refreshingly different, using thinking rather than brute repetitive 'grunt' work.

The instructor goes through the process and gives the body a signal to begin. Up it pops; Scout's attention transfers to the screaming and dancing, then the empty space when the body drops out of sight. He rockets out, leaping a log. Nothing happens at the body. I hold my breath while Scout dances around, the air filling with forest dust billowing up through shafts of light. Still nothing. He's getting frustrated: barking, dancing, pounding the ground with his paws, the forest ringing with his annoyance until he turns to me for help. I'm rooted to the spot. His eyes drag mine to the body. I call him. He hesitates, knowing the reward is with the body, always has been. It doesn't make sense, why would he come back to me? The air is charged, my fingernails dig into my palm. What will he do?

My command should override any desire he has. If he ignores me, I have a problem. Unsure what to do, Scout keeps glancing between me and the body. The instructor says call him. Scout steps towards me then stops and looks back at the body. I call again. A hand rests on my arm; the calm voice tells me to let Scout work it out. Scout barks at the body, then sprints back to me in frustration and annoyance. At my feet I tell him to speak; he bites my head off jumping so high I get the aroma of his breakfast. 'Show me,' I shout, waving my arms and moving forwards to the body. Scout barges past to bark again and again at the body, until I shout 'reward' and the body pops up, treat in hand for Scout to throw himself at. I am delirious, heaping praise.

Throughout the day we hone the return indication sequence, learning from each other what is good and what can be discarded. Like me, the Third

Man is so happy, our dogs too. Now the dogs can return and indicate, we've taken another step to the next assessment, the indication test, and from there, search training. Becoming operational suddenly feels within touching distance for us.

That evening we tell our local instructor the news. He tells us we can't train with the local handlers any more, that we're not ready to be doing the sequence. I'm silent. Training at night he says isn't safe; it will confuse the dog. I point out we train in daylight at weekends. The dog will be confused he says, take it or leave it.

Neither of us know what to do, it doesn't make sense, but our inexperience cannot argue. I talk it through with the instructor from that day; he can't understand the reasoning, but it's clear he does not feel able to be involved. If I want Scout to be a search dog, I must accept what the local instructor says.

Back home we revert to the tedium of our old training regime, the return indication sequence falling into disuse. I don't register the significance of this, about the thread that has spun out from my childhood and into my future.

It is Scout's first birthday. He is becoming a fine dog, with the quiet presence of one who is happy to inhabit his own space while a maelstrom rages around him. He is, like me, a loner. His character is thoughtful, stoic even. His nature is gentle. His intentions purposeful. He is fiercely protective of our bond and asks for nothing more than to be in my company. I am his family, his church.

Breeding has given him the white, black and tan markings that define the purity of his ancestry. Thick white socks cover large paws and thick pads, once pink, now black and scarred from working hard ground. The legs are covered in bristly white fur protecting the pink skin from thorns and ticks. Black and tan feathers drape from his body. A straight back holds a strong articulated torso cloaked in a dense glossy black coat that runs in waves to the long counterbalance tail. His chest is broad and shielded by a deep brilliant white waistcoat beneath which sits a downy thermal vest. The neck is circled by a luxuriously white Elizabethan ruff. The head is handsome, the face a chiaroscuro of tricolour markings, the long snout and bulbous nose lending him a comical air made only more certain by the thick pink tongue that habitually protrudes from soft leathery lips. The large pointy ears sit atop hooded tan eyebrows below which sit steady eyes. Dead centre of the forehead is a single white flash.

His disposition is pleasing. On first meeting he hesitates, unsure of his reception. Once confident he sidles up, turning his head in supplication like an errant member of a flock. By treats, soft words and tummy rubs, he measures a person's worth. The good and bad never forgotten.

Days are lengthening, helping me observe more detail in training. We've added a bark at the body when Scout finds them, sometimes teasing him with several barks until the reward appears. The treat is still a morsel of liver that doesn't please the bodies who are vegetarian, but keeps Scout engaged in the game. He's started barking when approaching the body, impressing me with his ability to work that out. Any thought of the return has stayed firmly at the Arctic training camp in Scotland.

Into spring I notice Scout is more lacklustre, almost as though he is going through the motions. At first, I think it must be me as I've grown frustrated at our pedestrian progress, pushing my thoughts down the lead to Scout. The Second Man and Third Man have moved on to using a toy as a reward, giving the game a huge shot of excitement. I'm chained to the liver, afraid to change what has worked.

I talk it over with our local instructor.

'Give me the treat,' pulling a ball out of his pocket.

He holds both to Scout who goes straight for the ball.

'There you are,' he says, 'bin the liver.'

It was that simple. Experience demonstrated what Scout valued most. I drop the liver like a hot potato, releasing a smile from Alison, and a hole in my wallet buying a ball on a rope.

We work with the high-octane, super-loud body we had in Brecon. Scout cannot get enough of her. He's unaware that she has the toy and is surprised when she pops up and the ball soars into the air, his wide eyes following its path until he catches it, falling to the ground, his mouth chewing on the rubber in pleasure. The body stays low, crawling on hands and knees across the tussocks, her hand reaching for the rope, teasing him. The ball is up in the air again; Scout catches it; the body grabs the rope and tugs, hard. Scout tugs back, the ball tight in his mouth, his eyes fixed on the body's eyes as they rock back and forth in rapture.

The bracken is shoulder high by summer, perfect for adding a second body, a decoy, hidden upwind at right angles to the pop-up body Scout will see. We let the decoy's scent build, crawling through the bracken stalks, lifting to the blanket of air that hangs above the patch of green fronds. It gets hot in a dense clump of bracken, lots of thermals developing, splitting scent and causing confusion. Scout does not know about the decoy.

A few weeks back I added in a new command. As I release Scout, I say 'find him out'. The body is 'him' – male or female it makes no difference to Scout. The command will be part of his operational trigger along with his work coat.

The pop-up body is a long way out on the moor. I wind Scout up, telling him they have his toy; as the body disappears, he strains against the lead, his cheeks puffing in and out, his eyes fixed on the pop-up location. 'Find him out!' Scout launches across the moor into the bracken; all I can see is the greenery parting as he makes his way through. Below the decoy is a thinner patch where I will be able to watch Scout's reaction as he enters the scent cone. If nothing, he will continue to the pop-up and get his reward. I'm holding my breath. His gangly legs power him forwards, eyes locked where the prize awaits. As he reaches the patch his nose snaps into the wind, the paws brake hard, grass and dirt spraying forwards, the back legs scrabbling as his body twists to the right, the legs gaining traction then ploughing him through the bracken, following the scent cells to the source until, moments later, I hear a bark and see his orange ball soar into the blue sky, followed by Scout rising out of the green sea, mouth wide open, eyes agog.

It is a beautifully big image. He's made the connection between scent and a human being more valuable than the body he saw and heard.

At home I go over the training session. I figure Scout must have registered human scent even with all those run-aways and pop-ups, he wasn't only relying on sight and sound. The decoy has demonstrated that scent is Scout's primary tool. His nose cut straight through the path of wind-borne human scent and his intelligence, knowledge and breeding turned him to the source.

I need to learn about the dark art of human scent.

We all smell.

Scent cascades from us; vast quantities of dead cells are shed from our skin and swirl around us like bits of torn leaf. Forty thousand micron-sized cells a minute, even when sleeping. The cells peel from skin, falling through clothing, dripping out of shirt cuffs and trouser bottoms, building towering clouds that billow from shirt collars and plume from the top of our heads. We litter the landscape. We leave clones of ourselves balanced finely on the ends of leaves. Place a hand on a rock – and there we are, long after we have gone. We can never leave no trace. It is our binary existence of human life. We were here. We are not.

Wind rustles scent into the earth's folds, piling like autumn leaves. Or it tumbles through a landscape like snowflakes on a winter wind, blown this way and that, catching a tree, settling on rock, or dirt, or blade of grass, spreading out from the human source in an ever-widening cone, marking our path and placing an anomaly in the landscape.

It is the anomaly Scout seeks. His forebears sought it in the mountains, on the high moorlands, deep in the wooded valleys. It is why I am here. For Scout, it is for the joy of an orange ball pitched high into a blue sky.

Most human scent comes from sweat glands, a concoction of chemicals, fats, vitamins and hormones, bound in a single cell pushed out into the world by our own thermal currents to catch on clothing, float to earth, place a breadcrumb trail to where we rest. Our heads are the most profligate. Great plumes of scent spewing off the top, an invisible smokestack of human pollution. Feet are next, all that sweat collecting in wool bound by thick leather and breathable plastic, then limbs, the torso, the groin, bits of human information continually flowing out like a stream of data.

As the cloud drifts from the source, cells clump together forming minute rafts, a flotilla of scent snagging on vegetation, landing softly on granite, surfing streams. In time forming an ever-widening triangle, the apex its source, the rest on and on, an infinity of human presence.

It is these scent notes that attract the attention of Scout. His nose – up to a hundred times more sensitive than a human nose – alerts him to the presence, somewhere, of a human. The scent snapping the nose into its flow, sampling data packets of life. It is a device designed for detecting scent. Long and thin with a constantly moist, absorbent tip, the long pink tongue smearing off samples. Inside it is riven with intricate galleries of hair and tissue moving scent into the olfactory chamber, the nerve centre. There it is analysed, catalogued and actioned, by a brain using half its complete processing power. The outcome: leave, follow or tell.

Weather plays a significant role in air-scenting searches; the understanding of it is crucial to effective dog handling. Rising thermal currents can pull scent from a valley floor, depositing it on a high summit. Likewise, a cooling thermal can pull scent down into the lower reaches of a landscape. Strong winds scatter scent far and wide. Heavy rains can wash scent away or collect it in pools. Snow can hold scent even in the depths of an avalanche.

The lie of the land, how time has shaped and shifted peat, rock and vegetation, affects how scent moves. Gullies collect, outcrops eddy, plains barrel, vegetation holds. Scent dumps are common. People stopping to rest saturate the location; many unsuspecting walkers and climbers have been found while enjoying a midday snack in a quiet place.

Scout still gets his reward from the body. The other two local dogs now train with the return indication sequence, but I'm told that we are not ready. I feel we are falling behind.

The problem I have is a thread running back to childhood. I want to please, be liked, do what I think people want me to do. Other than national training weekends, the local group is my only source of knowledge. Trust is becoming an issue. The reasons given for our lack of progress are never the same, often seem tenuous and do not reflect what I believe we can do. I'm beginning to question a lot of things and that is driving my mental health into an unstable place.

Alison asks to body one evening with the local dogs. She's noticed me getting frustrated and depressed; I reason Alison is wanting to support me, to let me know she is with me. After all, she's taking the brunt of the mood swings.

We gather in the early evening, Alison watching as handlers discuss their plans for training and bodies are allocated according to need. I say nothing, waiting to be told what to do. Alison is sent on to the moor to hide in the long grass with a radio so instructions can be given. We are going to work with the other two that have the return sequence. They go first. Find, return, indicate, guide. For Scout, Alison must pop up and get his attention then drop out of sight. Scout tears off on to the moor, barks at Mum, who springs up with his reward.

Alison erupts.

'Why isn't Scout allowed to do what the other two dogs are doing? He's just as good. Why is he being held back?'

'The instructor says he isn't ready.'

'Why isn't he? He's done exactly what the others have except return to you. They didn't find me straight away, Scout did. Why isn't he being allowed to progress?'

Alison presses the point at home, cuddling Scout as she vents. It's something so rarely seen in her that I'm taken aback. Her challenge is right, and true. The conflict is in me. Between not wanting to upset those I have placed my trust in and standing up for Scout.

That night in the darkness, I turn the conflict over in my mind, pulling at the same question again and again. Why can't we do the return indication sequence?

I enjoy the long journeys to national training camps. I'm taking my time to reach the deep south, stopping regularly to stretch both our legs, have a bite to eat. I listen to podcasts as I drive: adventure, literature, philosophy. Scout snoozes on layers of bedding he's pummelled until exactly right.

We arrive early, getting a bunk near a window, away from people, with a socket, and a clear path to the 2 a.m. and 4 a.m. toilet runs. I barricade myself in with rucksacks and bags, a tendency to sleepwalk bringing a fear of relieving myself across the bed of a hairy and very unhappy handler.

The derelict-looking bunkhouse is hunkered in a narrow cleft on Bodmin Moor. Two small boilers provide hot water; one is condemned. There is no heating. The shower has a granite floor with a hole for drainage; two copper pipes lead to ball valves acting as a mixer. A rust-spotted metal mirror sits on the windowsill. The shower door is the entrance door to the shower room and exits into a small kitchen; the door is wooden, unpainted, unvarnished. The lock does not work. The bunkroom is surprisingly comfortable with space to lay out kit and not be overlooked by too many neighbours. The single socket necessitates the use of multiple extension leads, brought from home by those with experience, which spread across the patchy linoleum floor like a mycelium. Into this are plugged phones, GPS units, Kindles, head torches, the odd electrical toothbrush – never a shaver. The appliances sprout like mushrooms as more people arrive. Inevitably there comes a time when the whole system reaches overload and the single fifty-amp fuse trips. Power is restored when the offending appliance has been removed, usually after much argument as to who plugged what in last. Cooking is carried out using the four rings or the single oven fed by propane gas. Or one of the two microwaves, but only if everything else is switched off, including the tower fridge and freezer. If this is not done cries of anguish fill the building as the half-frozen ready meal still has a coating of frost. There are better-appointed bothies in the remotest areas of Scotland. The bunkhouse is perfect.

I find the national instructor and explain we should be doing the return indication sequence. He agrees. I feel vindicated. For the first time I feel that I do know enough about the training to challenge what I am being told to do. Pleased I've stood up for Scout, I say nothing to the handler who has been instructing me back home, and sleep well.

Next morning, the national instructor sets up an exercise for Scout. Scout finds the body and waits. The body remains still. The trainer tells me to call Scout back. Scout returns and I tell him to speak, he barks, I tell him to 'show me' and begin walking to the body. Scout digs the return indication sequence from Aviemore out of his mind and muscle memory and runs the loop until I get there, and the body pops up with the reward. We practise all morning, away from the other dogs, refining the timing, taking out any spare seconds so it is seamless. By midday we have a return indication sequence. I guess hell hath no fury like that of a mother.

Over the weekend we add two further elements. Until now, Scout has always seen the body leave him with his toy, a grown adult skipping across a moor swinging a ball on a piece of rope while squealing in a high-pitched voice. It's hard to ignore. From now on Scout will not see or hear the bodies. He will have to find them and run the return indication sequence. I will know where the body is in case something goes awry, and Scout needs a little help. Errorless training. The second element is a twist. I now have Scout's reward toy, which he does not know … yet.

The first time we try it Scout is confused. Where is the screaming human with his toy? He remains still, looking at me then out to the silent moor. The instructor tells me to let Scout work it out. We walk; Scout keeps checking me. My back begins to lock up with tension, my teeth grind. I emit a low growl to get Scout to leave and find the body. He thinks I'm angry. I lighten my voice, shake my shoulders, become aware the instructor is a few steps behind, watching. I smile and tell Scout to 'find him out'. When other handlers say this their dogs shoot off like greyhounds. Scout looks more anxious, his confusion threatening him. Maybe it is too soon.

I keep up a steady progression through the scent cone of the body. Time has helped us; the scent pool seeping across the moor is strong. Scout's nose snaps into the cone, ears prick up; he springs into the long grass, surfing through the waves of yellow stalks until he is lost to me. A bark, then Scout on the incoming wave to my feet, a bark, a spin around, and back he goes. I'm running as fast as I can trying to stay upright and in sight of him. The body is there, Scout standing off looking at me, barking. I release the toy into the air; his eyes widen into dark pools, tracking its trajectory then launching to intercept it mid-flight. As he crashes down the body pops up to grab the toy and begin a game of vigorous tug, both trying to prise the prize from each other, rocking backwards and forwards, Scout's tail wearing away the grass behind him. It's the best reward he's ever had.

· · ·

The local instructor feels we still need the body to perform a pop-up before Scout is released, so now we add that to the return indication sequence and go over it again and again. Scout loves it. So much so, he becomes addicted to this crack cocaine of dog training – just one more run, then just one more. He must realise that I've got the ball, so why run to where the screaming person is? Just bark at Dad for the reward. Simple. I'm too slow to pick up what is happening until the habit is firmly ingrained in Scout's psyche. We are getting close to a fork in the path of our training. I will choose the hardest route. It will change everything.

His mind is locked in now, barking incessantly, pounding the ground in front of me demanding his reward. It becomes a battle of wits, of sleepless nights and growing stress. Handlers offer advice but nothing works, the grain going deeper, and I can see no way out. I'm unhappy, the problem consuming my every moment. I'm unpleasant to be around at home, all our dogs keeping well out of my way, the slightest upset firing off my hair-trigger anger.

I begin isolating at local training, keeping away from the others, trying anything to get Scout to leave me. They leave me alone, focus on their own needs; I'm not their problem. Each time I think we are making progress and rejoin the main group, only for Scout to fail to leave again, and back we go to the cooler, so we don't disrupt the others, suiting everyone. I imagine them thinking we won't get back on track. Another dog won't leave the body to return to its handler. The quick correction underlines my continued failure. All this passes down the lead to Scout – the more frustrated I get the greater the tension, the more I fail the more despondent I become. A vicious spiral taking us further away from our goal.

It all crashes down one bright Sunday morning on the beautiful Ramsley Moor. I'm back in the local group, nervous but hopeful. Scout has a body a hundred metres from the green track we stand on. I work on his motivation, telling him over and over to 'find him out', telling him he will get his toy. As I release him after the pop-up, he begins his bark and dance routine. I try hard to keep it light, aware handlers are watching. Finally, he moves off, only for his attention to be taken by another dog running across him. He comes back to me barking, digging in with his paws for a long session. In my stressed-out state I'm furious; dogs are supposed never to interfere with another's training run. I explode at the local instructor whose dog has transgressed, telling him what's the point of training if his dog is going to ruin it. 'Well, fuck off then,' is his answer, and walks on.

I stand stunned, watching his back move away from me. Scout is cowering. I walk off in silence, Scout on the lead, passing the handlers at the gate who remain quiet, refraining from eye contact. At home I shatter into pieces, traumatised, nerves shredded, convinced we are at the end of our journey. It's a despairingly dark moment.

As the dust settles, I get a call, checking I'm all right, from one of the handlers who saw what happened. I'm touched by this. My big worry is training: should I tough it out and stay with the local group?

I say, for whatever reason, something isn't right between me and that local instructor. It's unstable, lacks consistency, and has a negative impact on me and Scout. When I've tried to discuss it, concerns are dismissed. At times, the relationship improves only to disintegrate with no warning or reason. I've put my faith in a person, but it hasn't worked. I'm aware I'm not alone in having these problems, and that there may be reasons that have nothing to do with me. But it's my responsibility to sort it out. But how? I could always train with the other group local to me; it's more travelling and I've never had any contact with them, but what other options do I have? The handler knows both groups and feels the group I have been training with is a better choice. But it's my decision.

I'm aware of friction between the two groups: personalities, difference in techniques. It isn't uncommon, the whole of mountain rescue has its factions. Occasionally, squabbles break out as a group grapples for control in the belief their way is the best. At the extreme it leads to areas going it alone. More usually the verbal jousting eases back into mutual antipathy. I stay out of politics and personal arguments, knowing such eruptions eventually settle down, everything returning to how it was. But this I cannot fix. I've tried, but my trust has evaporated. Painfully, I step away from the group. We are in the wilderness.

I write walking guidebooks. A by-product of my fall, my first piece of writing was a blog trying to understand what happened that day. It got picked up by a few online magazines, and shortly after I got the opportunity to write about walking in the Peak District, books and magazine articles. Without any planning I had a writing career.

Now Scout is old enough to stretch his legs, he accompanies me on my research trips, which builds his stamina and strength. He's still all limbs and corners, but his manners are impeccable; the walks give him experience of new environments and challenges. Working out how to get over stiles is his first big learning curve. Ladder stiles he eventually works out, though hearing his elbows clattering against the wood has me wincing. Kissing gates confuse him, not understanding where he should be. He gets there in the end, working out he needs to wait, for a kiss. The hard ones are squeeze stiles – it's apparent he has no sense of his size in a space. Some he goes through, others he gets stuck. If I stand back, give him time and encouragement, he will analyse a problem, try a few solutions until one succeeds, keeping it in his memory bank. When confronted with something new, he works an algorithm until something fits.

The next guidebook takes me to the softer limestone and pasture country of the Peak District. The sheep are so comfortable around us they come for a chat about whatever sheep and Border collies chat about. The walking is gentle, the landscape unfolding peacefully before us. We spend time sitting and watching. Resting against walls warmed by the sun, or in the shade of a tree in the heat of the day, Scout resting his chin on my legs, the occasional snack snaffled, a post-dinner snooze descending on us. It is a magical time moulding us together. The break clears away the rubble of recent events, enabling me to see the building blocks that are needed to continue.

Somewhere, Scout has got stuck on not leaving me. I suspect the repetitive local training, and even though I was following advice, ultimately it was my responsibility to guide Scout's development. Whenever I have been in situations like this I have reverted to basics, no matter what the issue is. Then I rebuild from the very beginning, hoping to spot where I went wrong, and erase that from the future. We go back to Hillsborough Park and begin with obedience, correcting any issues that have crept into Scout's response. Working on the sports field, we run through the various stages. When each step is consolidated we move on.

It's the height of summer and the park is full of children, picnickers and the ice cream van. Scout becomes a bit of a celebrity; a little fan club of parents and children stands looking as we go through our routine. The big finale is the down stay out of sight. People set watches, film him on their phones, comment on what he might be thinking. Some ask why we train, the respect for Scout clear in their eyes. Usually, a child will approach with an ice cream, the vanilla running down their hand as they wobble across the grass with their gift for Scout, who, first lick, has it out of their hand. By the third lick it's gone and Scout is sniffing the child's hands, licking fingers, the child squealing delight. These are moments that take the sting out of the last months. When it all fell apart, I thought we'd had something taken from us that was good. Now I think it will be much better.

I've explained to national instructors what we are doing, and they all support my action. We no longer train with local handlers, but still attend national training camps. I need to heal my wounds in isolation. The two handlers we began training with are progressing smoothly and moving well ahead of us now. I've never seen it as a competition, staying pragmatic in the ups and downs, focusing on my own responsibilities. One of the local handlers says my plan seems to be working and not to stop just to placate others. Of all the handlers he's the one I respect the most, getting on calmly with the job, not playing politics, focusing on what he and his dog need. I'm sure he's aware of the last months. He was there when it all came apart on that beautiful moor, and registered my stoic response when perhaps others would have taken a different path. His reaching out has a profound effect on me. I can choose my own path; there are people who do want us to succeed. I tell Alison about this flicker of hope, and for the first time in many months we feel we have a future.

I need to rebuild the return indication sequence, the bit that eventually broke down. To do this I need a body. I could ask one of the local bodies, but they will be needed for the other dogs, and I don't want to deplete resources. And we need somewhere to train that isn't a sports field.

Following our experience of the crack cocaine of pop-ups I'm wary of using Alison all the time in case we end up creating another addiction for Scout. But Alison could work once a week if I can get a few more people to add variety.

A few minutes from home, quiet Loxley Common is perfect for our needs. Normally, training requires the permission of the landowner. This is council land, so it's owned by the people of the city, the 'commoners', me, looked after by the commoners and the council. I don't ask permission. The mix of terrain – woodland, heathland, crag, boulder field, open areas and copse – is a microcosm of the type of landscape we will operate in. The only thing it does not have is significant ascent, which is not an issue at present. There is no need for long drives, so more time at home and less stress.

A bench and table become our Office. We keep the distance between Scout and Alison close, getting lots of joy for Scout. A little obedience work to begin, ringing the changes each time so we do not create a habit, then three runs on Alison, pop-up or run away, other times Alison hiding for Scout to search. I have the reward toy. Everything ends with a find and a massively overdone reward, lots of squealing, tugging and Scout diving around for his reward. When we finish, we rest enjoying the summer evening, with the view of the city bathed in golden light. Alison brings a little picnic, and Scout gets us all to himself.

Some days, I take a pack of clothes waiting to be washed, hide it on the Common during the day, a pinned note asking people to leave it be. I shove it between boulders, hang it from trees, ram it under heather. A few hours later the scent will have built, the cone moving a good distance from the source. I'm interested to see what Scout will do when he enters the cone either when working or just as part of a walk. It's a great game, allowing me to adjust action on the move, sometimes guiding Scout slowly and calmly to explore the location, other times walking him across the scent cone to see his reaction when the scent hits his nose. Gradually, I extend distance and time, working longer before the find is made.

I've stumbled across an important tool when looking for a missing person. Personal items – a dropped set of keys, a discarded phone, clothing – can indicate the presence of a missing person in the locale, or that they have passed through that point. I don't want Scout to bring it to me, I want him to take me to it. That way I can make a thorough search of the area.

We're enjoying our home schooling so much it's showing at monthly national camps; our development has stabilised into a steady progression. Now, I need a body at home to mirror what we are doing on the national courses. I post a request on social media for help, saying that the role is mainly lying down on cold muddy ground for long periods of time, the legs becoming numb, then being assailed by a barking dog and having to play vigorously. It's fun.

We are deluged with offers and Paul joins our little training camp. This one man's kindness changes everything. He's never been a body, so I teach him, analysing the process to get the outcome I need, catapulting my knowledge beyond anything I had imagined. Playing ball gets Scout and Paul used to each other and quickly we move on to run-aways and pop-ups. Change one thing at a time is advice I've been given. As Paul and Scout bond I reduce Alison's presence until she isn't there at all.

After a few weeks we drop pop-ups and run-aways. Now, body Paul hides before Scout and I step on to the Common, letting his scent accumulate and drift. At my radio signal he shouts for Scout, giving him an audible beacon. It works, Scout completing the return indication sequence even as I increase distance and time. After months of hard work, we discard the beacon and Scout is on his own. There is no more bark and dance routine, he heads straight out with purpose. We are back on track.

. . .

October brings the Peak District national training camp. We are at Heatherdene in the Upper Derwent Valley, finding bodies hidden in dense undergrowth or behind pine trees in a large woodland. We work blind, neither of us knowing where the bodies are. This is the meat and bones of operational search call-outs, finding the unknown in the unknown.

We're given the defined boundaries of a search area, a boulder, a fallen tree, a drystone wall, the track we stand on. I'm not sure I have correctly identified the right tree amid hundreds of others; I try to retain details but once we move into a space, perspective changes, that small rock becomes a big boulder. Now that Scout has the return indication sequence firmly embedded in muscle and mind, training has shifted from him to me.

Late morning, we are pulled away from the training group for an indication test. We're relaxed and understand the boundaries we are given. This is a well-known woodland for me, the landmarks easy to hold in my mind. We'll walk down the track cutting across a firm wind blowing up to us. The indication test assesses Scout's ability to detect scent, find the body, return to me, tell me and take me to the body. Scout is a few metres ahead, trotting along nicely, the instructor a few metres behind me. Scout's nose whips to the right and he charges through the brash, weaving through trees, skittles to a halt behind a large trunk, barks, returns to me, barks, spins around and sets off back to the trunk, me following behind. When I get there the body is smiling, Scout is smiling, I'm smiling. 'Good boy,' I shout and launch his reward. We head back to the track and move towards the stop point a few hundred metres away. By the time we reach it Scout has found three bodies and indicated each one. I don't know how many there are. I'm asked if we have found everyone. I say yes.

'You've passed.'

That's it. We progress on. The months of being in the wilderness are over.

Would I change anything about these past six months? It would have been good to have avoided the trauma, no one needs that in their day. I guess the important lessons will gradually become clear as time works its magic. For now, I've learned I know more than I realise and can trust my instincts. I've learned to listen, evaluate, take what I need and discard the rest, no matter how many dogs the adviser has trained. I've learned to change one thing at a time, consolidate, move on. I've learned that people with the best advice aren't necessarily the ones with the loudest voice, but sometimes they are. That the ones I think are least approachable are the ones who will reach out a hand. But not always. That often I am right, and Scout is never wrong.

Life away from training moves on. Alison's been lecturing at the university's Wuhan campus in China. My fellow students on my creative writing degree tease me, asking what it was like before mobile phones. Nicer, I reply. They can't believe I do maths in my head, having the answer before they have opened their app. I see the value an education can give, and I'm saddened by a life in silent acquiescence.

Call-outs are the obligatory mountain bikers. There are searches for missing walkers and runners, and an increasing number of vulnerable people. Austerity has pushed the vulnerable to the margins of a failing welfare system. Many with mental health needs are finding help harder to access and cry out for help. Mountain rescue uses its special skills, and ability to work at night to find vulnerable people.

At the onset of winter, it's time for my core skills assessment: rope, search and navigation. The search is simple, but it's surprising how many people fail to spot the mobile phone on a fence post, or the fully clothed dummy hanging in a tree. For a dog this isn't an issue, but humans must switch their brains to search mode to avoid missing something of importance. Rope assessment involves working with ropes, knots, gear and abseils, everything I spend limited time with and my weakest area. I pass, but criticise myself for going too fast and making silly mistakes. The navigation assessment I love. This winter it is on the featureless Saddleworth Moor high on the Pennines, at night. In two hours, I must find five brown sticks, two-and-a-half centimetres square, sticking out of the ground no more than thirty centimetres, each a check point on a five-kilometre course. Each checkpoint is given as a ten-figure grid reference giving me a one-metre square to hit. Only a paper map and a compass are allowed. Scout cannot accompany me due to his ability to detect human scent on the markers, leading me straight to them. After several days of heavy snow, the clag has come down and reduced visibility to less than two metres; thankfully there is no windchill, making it a pleasant night walk. I find all five in good time. I have a great time, despite going up to my waist in icy cold water hiding beneath snow drifts. When I'm finished my quickest exit back to control is over a fence and along the road. The fence gives way as I throw myself over, dumping me head first into the roadside ditch filled with snow, ice, old beer cans and slime. I'm incredibly happy.

I've left my hand torch behind. It will be a good opportunity to check Scout's progress. In the morning, we set out across the moor. The wind has picked up, pushing us around on the hard snow and ice, but the visibility is good. Scout is ahead, sweeping on to high ground. He gets the scent across the wind, his jack-knifed body following his nose in and out of a couple of deep peat groughs (channels), through some small drifts, until he vanishes. Silence. I keep on his track until he's back and indicates for me to scramble on to high ground and follow. I see him on an ice sheet by the wooden peg, my torch by his feet, tail swishing, pleased as punch with himself. I love it. We have lots of ball play, his first time on ice and he can't quite understand why he's sliding all over the place. We spend half an hour playing on the moor, throwing the ball, me hiding, him running along frozen streams, keeping us warm. The torch still works.

My team has introduced a fitness challenge, the shape of some members showing a great fondness for fry-ups. Like many teams in the country the age profile is heavily slanted toward the upper end, and some are reaching the lower limit of their ability to sustain a presence on the hill. It's a six-kilometre route with 300 metres of ascent along an ancient track over the high moors. It must be done in ninety minutes. I take sixty-four minutes; Scout wins, probably covering twice the distance.

Handlers are practitioners of a dark art, held together by rituals and lucky charms, convinced without them they will lose the seemingly tenuous grasp on success. The reward is a major focus – a toy kept only for that purpose, special food, a pungent dried fish is popular – trigger words, 'find him out'. Rituals are big, the rucksack always packed the same way, radio in a particular spot, the same clothing worn, the working dog coat slipped on at a precise moment.

By happenstance, on the first day of the next national training weekend I find a way to increase the value of Scout's reward. To help Scout after he'd overcome rock and dense vegetation high up in the clouds to find the body who was reluctant to engage, I go into overdrive, tugging the rope of his toy while he bites down harder and tugs back further. This swings both the ball and Scout violently, his legs waltzing through the air. Scout grips tighter, the tug of war setting his eyes on fire. The eyes never leave mine, a wide smile grows across his face, the lips flap as he swings back and forth, ears fly out, a low growl leaks out between teeth, his body ripples with joy. I am so deep in play I begin to growl like Scout which makes him pull harder and growl louder. At the next find he is eager to get me to the location, running back and forth several times, complaining all the while at my sloth. We play the game again, the body looking on in astonishment. If I could get the bodies to do this, Scout would have the time of his life. I need a suitable candidate.

The next day, after the morning briefing, I catch up with our body for the day, a young prospective handler eager to please. In training, each handler explains how the dog should be rewarded. Any unusual instructions are demonstrated, usually how to play with the toy or interact with the dog. Some are simple, others get complicated, it all depends how mad the handler is. I go through the procedure.

'To maintain Scout's progress, I've increased the value of his reward. We tried it yesterday and it works really well. I'll show you what to do when I give the reward command.'

'OK.'

The other handlers begin to form a circle around the three of us, arms folded, settling in for the entertainment.

'When I give the command, have a good game of tug with Scout, be as rough as you want, he likes that so really go for it.'

'Are you sure? I don't want to hurt him.'

Scout follows the ping pong of the conversation, his ears pricking up when he hears his name, the eyebrows rising as his toy swings into view. I give Scout the ball toy and we tug it between us, swinging him around, all four limbs splayed in the air, eyes fixed on the prize, bared teeth around his beloved toy.

'That's how he likes it.'

'OK.'

'There is one more element, and this is crucial. You must "Grrrr".'

I can feel the handlers desperate to see where this goes.

'Grrrr?'

'Yes. "Grrrr." Try it.'

'Are you having me on? Is this some initiation test to be a handler?'

'You might think it's a test. I am deadly serious.'

The audience, now swollen, stalling the exodus to training, wants a demonstration. So, I play tug with Scout and I 'Grrrr'. Scout is clearly loving it, and that confuses the body, their confidence undermined by the acquiescence of the audience and the joy of Scout.

'There. That's what Scout needs. The "Grrrr" is the most important bit of his reward, it winds him high. Look at his little face. Look how happy he is.

How could you not want to make a dog with a face like that the happiest dog on the hill? How cruel would it be to deny him his one little pleasure?'

'If this is a wind-up, I'm going to batter you.'

Ball in hand, the body, with a final look back at smirking handlers, teases Scout with the ball, his paws dancing, his bark ringing.

'I just know this is going to come back and bite me.'

The dogsbody, full marks, puts everything into it. Scout is in search dog heaven. The attention, the movement, the sounds, everything is pure unadulterated joy. As the body pulls and swings, they emit a loud stream of 'Grrrrs', both lost in the game.

'I'm knackered. I can't speak. My throat is raw.'

'Yes. That happened to me.'

The 'Grrrr' is born.

2018

The next stage of development is clearing an area efficiently. 'Clearing' is the term used for searching ground using the dog and the wind to catch any human scent should it be there. 'Efficiently' means clearing without the handler walking over every inch of land and peering behind every boulder, saving time and energy, allowing the dog to find a human should they be there, or search managers to move their focus elsewhere should no human be present.

The key to clearing an area efficiently is the collecting boundary. This is the edge of a search area that the wind is blowing to, and as follows, carrying any scent in its path. Beginning from the collecting boundary and working toward the opposite boundary will give the dog its best opportunity of detecting human scent.

It is the skill of the handler that now comes to the fore, working the dog to ensure the ground is cleared. Time is extended slowly, building up to a two-hour search, which demands fitness and concentration from both handler and dog. It is not something that comes overnight. Operationally, the dog team can be working for many hours in appalling conditions; resilience is a key tool in the kit. To achieve this the dog team must be put under conditions that maximise time, fitness and weather conditions. This normally takes between twelve and eighteen months.

At the end of the period of training the team will be assessed in five areas over three days in mountainous terrain in winter, or close to winter conditions.

. . .

Winter roars in with the Beast from the East, bringing heavy snowfall, gale-force winds and below-freezing temperatures. The storm strikes quickly, trapping motorists, bringing down power lines, cutting communications. Thankfully, few people venture out on to the hill, though the team is on high alert. I'm manning the social media platform, taking note of conditions and feeding back any problems with the roads from our Land Rover that has been out and about. There are many.

Our base high in the South Pennines gets the full force of any weather from the west, east or north, as do the roads that criss-cross the moors, the small settlements in the valleys and the remote farmsteads that cling to the sides. It's a magical landscape in winter; snow removes the drystone walls leaving just contours of smoothed icing. It can be harsh. That same smoothness whips up the wind and snow, freezing anything in its path. Iced roads out of the valleys quickly seal communities off. Across Britain teams are rescuing motorists stranded on motorways as village halls are commandeered to accommodate humans who never expected not to reach their destination.

As I pump out information I get messages from stranded people. We rescue a lorry driver on a steep Pennine hill, his brakes frozen solid, no food or drink, and no warmth. A woman needs hospital treatment, but the ambulance cannot get to the remote farm; we rescue her and transfer her to grateful paramedics waiting on the half-cleared highway. An overturned vehicle is checked out and found to be empty; a search of the immediate area has no sign of people. Local media arranges to film us at our base; news outlets call for information and images. For three days I play tennis with global media from my study while the team check on abandoned vehicles, deliver groceries and medications, ensure the old and infirm are in good fettle, and help anyone in distress. When the Beast finally subsides, the team has been working for a solid seventy-two hours.

The storm abated, Scout and I head to the gritstone edges. He's never experienced deep snow, so I'm interested to see how he fares. Our route takes us up an old hollow way, the twisted black branches of ancient oaks arching beneath a vivid blue sky, the trees bedecked with lines of white powder until the sun springs them free. There's virgin snow deep enough to rise above my boots and more. Scout loves it, his body moving smoothly over the surface until he finds a big curving drift to plunge into head first, popping out glowing with snow and a big smile. We play in the deep powder, bounding across snow-capped heather moguls sinking into great hollows of snow, each taking turns to pull the other free. It is a time full of fun and togetherness.

With Alison and all the dogs, we climb to the top of Win Hill. At the trig pillar, the view across the snow-laden Peak District is wonderful. Even though there's a windchill there are plenty of people taking in the scenery, most in hard winter kit, barring two young men in T-shirts. I say nothing but mark their route off the hill just in case.

I've slowed down in training, taking time to set up each exercise, paying attention to what is around me, which way the wind blows, temperature, time, our mood and energy. I make detailed notes after each session, thoughts on what worked and what didn't, any unforeseen problems or nice surprises. It's part confidence, part development, highlighting threads that run through the sessions. It shows me that if I give Scout too many commands it confuses him, his frustration brought out in dancing and barking. Now after the initial command I stay quiet, allow him to get on with his job. He does, working things out his way. It shines a light on what happens when we introduce something new, a body high in a tree perhaps to simulate a climber stuck on a crag or a suicide. If we go straight into the find, the process begins to unravel; Scout gets mixed messages that confuse his algorithm. If we break it down into small steps and gradually reconnect established skills to the new bits, the process rebalances and runs smoothly. This focus on each component of a scenario is a feedback loop regenerating each iteration.

Scout is two years old and almost fully grown. His body needs to fill out and he still has moments of puppy madness. His limbs and joints have knitted together well, all those five-minutes-per-month-of-age walks paying dividends. He's becoming bolder in his approach to the landscape; crags and water hold no fear for him nor does snow and rain. His only dislike is bramble which spikes his pads, and bracken that can suffocate him in the humidity. At home he's still the incomer with our other dogs, Monty and Olly, and for now, has decided to let it go, happy in our world and special times together. He spends a lot of house time simply watching what happens, content being a loner.

Scout's return indication is extraordinarily strong, with a distinctive, defined quality. When he finds a person, he comes straight back with a purpose, eyes full of intent, moving inexorably to me, his face telling me he has a find. At my feet, his head lifts and emits a single loud bark from a mouth so wide I can see the bottom of his throat, spins around and returns to the body using the exact same line, over boulders, across gullies, repeating everything until I reach the body and he has his reward. It is unequivocal and I have complete faith in what he is saying. It's a major psychological step. If trust is not present confidence can ebb away; a handler may look to second-guessing where a body might be rather than clearing the area. Good handlers build that trust step by step, through failure and frustration, using kindness, patience and perseverance, coming out the other side as a fine search dog team.

We have deep snow on the ground. It's a beautiful night, a deep blue sky pricked with stars, a full moon drifting shadows across the Common, the day's snow folding in waves, running along blackened boughs, smoothing the hardness of gritstone. The land holding its breath, waiting.

Body Paul is by the Ordnance Survey triangulation pillar, in place a good thirty minutes before we begin our search. I know where he is. I am wanting a long search through woodland on a cold night with deep snow on the ground and trees heavy with sparkling snowflakes, to see how conditions affect Scout working. A westerly pushes freezing air towards us, letting Scout pick up Paul's scent as it creeps through trees, piles against walls, settles in hollows. Paul has approached from the west; the ground has no evidence of him as we work from the east, other than the scent-laden air. He's wrapped in many layers of clothing – hats, gloves, a bivvy bag, a sleeping bag and several mats – decanting his scent to form a pool around him before beginning its eastward journey. When Scout finds him, Paul will say 'dog in' over the radio to let me know. It's the only safety line I hold. The errorless training.

Training on my own has given me freedom to develop strategies without being blown off course by someone's advice, collecting live data, turning theory and hypothesis into practice.

'Body Paul in position.'

Scout begins getting ready for work, the van rocking with excitement at Paul's trigger. I open the doors, finding him pushing forwards, plant kisses on his forehead to hold him, put his work coat on. He knows all the triggers now, his mind in work mode before paws are on the ground. Put my pack by the house door, there he is waiting. Make a flask of tea, he'll go to where his coat hangs.

I brief him, telling him to take his time and have fun, but not to take any chances jumping from boulder to boulder in the deep snow. He looks over my shoulder at the whiteness beyond. We take a moment to absorb everything. It is so gorgeous, a Christmas card, there is even a Christmas tree bedecked in shiny ornaments on the heath. Scout sniffs the air, pecking at the shadows. The dog walkers have gone home, the cold has beaten off partying youth, wildlife has bedded down or turns in a warm burrow during the long winter hibernation. Silence beneath an endless sky.

The wind runs a diagonal from the Atlantic, over the Pennines. It barrels down the valley on to the Common where it weaves through ash, oak and silver birch, heather, bracken and moss, over drystone walls, races around numerous small quarries, lifts to mark boulders, the remaining scent moving through man and dog, and onwards down streets, rattling the windows and doors of the city bunkered down for the night, each molecule carrying the data of an existence.

Scout keeps a steady sweep up to my eyes watching for the command; I stoop and kiss him, holding my cheek close to his, feeling the warmth of his fur and the cold pricks of snow melting a line down my skin. As I switch his light on, I whisper, asking if he's going to find Paul. His ears spring up, and he leans forwards letting me slip his lead. Free now, he dances and barks letting the tension wash out of him. 'Find him out.' I wave him off, he moves a few metres, stops, dances. Another command to find Paul, then I'm quiet. Scout loosens off muscle and brain, like a runner shaking legs while giving total focus to the finish line. This as part of our set-up, his process of resolving any inner conflict.

I was once told that I might have to get stern with Scout if this palaver at the beginning continues, grab him by his ruff and rant into his face. I'm told other handlers had to do this and it worked. I've heard of some 'taking the dog behind a shed', a euphemism to show the handler is boss; others have used a rubber hose across the dog's nose when they are having sheep worrying issues, 'de-sheeping' they call it, an old shepherd's trick they say. For us, the loud 'no' has been enough.

Looking across the whiteness, I map out the land with my mind, and ignore his protestations. Eventually he gets tired of being ignored and moves off, skipping over the compacted snow and ice, dissolving into the woodland.

Working my way towards the wall that separates the Common from the woodland, I hear Scout's bark split the night. He cannot possibly have had time to find Paul. I haven't had a 'dog in' either. Scout thunders through the opening straight to me; everything about him shouts *find*. I can see the excitement in his eyes piercing through the darkness, see it rippling along his body. As he breaks the snow in front of me his head lifts and a mighty bark rattles trees; he spins, retraces his steps without once looking behind, and merges once more into the trees.

He must have found Paul.

Another bark, another burst out of the trees. He's so consumed by his find he slides into my feet, snow-ploughing ahead of him. He indicates, shoots me a frustrated look and is gone.

He really has found Paul.

I pick up the pace, noting the look he gave – me letting the team down – and slip through the wall into the heavy silence of the woodland. I stand and listen, allowing senses to adjust in the monochrome landscape, sweeping my eyes through the trees, scanning nature's barcode, my head torch strobing against trunk and snow. I can see a light, Scout's I assume, for who else would be here, only mad men and English dogs. The light moves through the trees blinking on and off, there and not there, a binary existence. It's Scout, heading back to me, intensely angry, the bark and then away again. I feel slow as he draws me down into the dense nothingness where the trees are thickest, and the boulders huddle in crowds. I scramble across rocks, testing snow-covered gaps for leg breakers, my hands freezing.

The light ahead of me has ceased its movement. My directions to Paul must have been poor; this is a long way from the trig pillar. I'm close enough to see Scout watching me, see his displeasure, tapping his back paw and glancing at a watch. I apologise, saying I'm trying to be careful. He disappears behind a large holly tree. Finally, I reach the track he was impatiently waiting on. Scout sits in the centre of the broad white strip, his tail scouring scallop shells in the snow, his head to one side, eyes searching for his toy. There's just me and Scout and falling snow.

I ask him to show me; his head turns left. I move a step closer. He looks back at me then to the left again. Two more steps and I'm beside him. He looks at me then side glances left, the whites filling the space. Almost blending with the snow-covered holly are two people clinging to each other, their eyes darting between me and Scout, their faces full of fear.

'Good boy.'

Scout springs into the air as I launch his toy; I grab the rope and he pulls me to the ground where I flail around issuing lots of 'Grrrr'. In my periphery, I see the two people, male and female, arms around each other trying to step further back, the holly making them jump as it pricks through their clothing, showers of snow dumping on to their heads. I notice they don't have many clothes on – no coat, no winter layers, no hat or gloves – more suited for a night on the dance floor, the thin white tops glowing blue from my headlamp. It's odd, this time of year, at night when it's snowing.

'Are you okay?'

'We're lost. We're trying to get out of the wood. That dog kept coming up to us and barking and running away.'

'This is Scout. He's training to be a search dog and you two are his first real find. Where are your coats?'

'We got lost. We can't find our way out, we're very cold. Can you help us?'

I'm on a massive high and almost forget the hero of the moment who is nodding at his ball for more play. I am so proud of him, finding someone in distress, doing his job.

On the way off the Common I ask if I can take a photo, excited words tumbling from my mouth, the air condensing around our heads in a cloud. I'll put it on social media, it's such a big thing for Scout. No, they say, no to names, no to address, no to phone number, they just want to get home. We guide them to the lights of civilisation, their heads together exchanging whispers. I watch, the strangeness coalescing around my mind. Why would anyone come out on a night like this wearing so little? We stand side by side watching the two become dots in the cityscape. I wonder if Scout knows what he's done. I tell him he did good and give him a treat. Then remember poor Paul who must be freezing.

Working through the wood I watch to see when Scout first detects Paul. Two hundred metres from the trig pillar Scout's head snaps in its direction, nose sampling and analysing. Then he is gone. *The strike.* Scout has entered the scent cone of a human. 'Dog in.' The signal from Paul that Scout has found him. Soon, Scout is back at my feet with the perfect indication. This time he doesn't need to lose patience with me, the ground is easy; as I reach the trig I shout 'good boy' and launch his toy as Paul rises, snow sliding off his bivvy bag. He warms up playing ball. I can see how much Scout finding him is a thousand times more valuable than the find thirty minutes ago; he is so happy.

I tell Paul about Scout's find, and how the couple were dressed. Neither of us can work it out.

There is a possibility the speed limit may not have been adhered to on the short drive home. I burst into the house yelling for Alison to tell her about Scout's find. He's showered with more love and more treats, Monty and Olly joining in the dancing that breaks out in the kitchen.

Alison tucks Scout into bed covering him in more kisses. A shower eases the electricity running through my body while my mind reruns the exercise, playing over the odd response of the couple. The penny drops.

Scout's find is splashed across social media, picked up by the papers, making the front page of the *Daily Telegraph*, Scout's beautiful face beaming out from several columns. The BBC phone, wanting Scout on *The One Show* that evening, along with the two people rescued. I say I don't think that will be possible.

'Why? It's a great story, and Scout is so beautiful.'

'It is, he is. But they didn't want any publicity.'

'Why? They must have been so relieved and happy Scout saved them.'

'Probably. But I don't think they would want it known.'

'We'd be very gentle.'

'I'm not explaining myself very well. I don't think they should have been there, at night, not wearing many clothes, with each other.'

'Really. Oh. Ooooh, I see what you mean. Does that happen a lot?'

'It's Scout's first time, but I'm told it's not unusual.'

'Fantastic. What a shame. It would have been great to have such a handsome dog on the show.'

Our fifteen minutes of fame slips by. I'm glad. It would have brought too much attention. Aside from the comedy of it all, Scout did his job well, and I trusted his judgement. In the following days I bask in the moment and Scout absorbs the praise heaped on him from the community on the Common. We never see or hear from the couple again.

The months of solitary training are paying off. We have a solid indication and Scout understands his role. Our challenge now is to work larger areas and tougher ground to get us ready for operational assessment. We need higher, steeper terrain that is complicated with streams, crags, boulder fields, deep gullies and dense woodland. Ground that is difficult and demanding to operate in mentally and physically, for both of us. I need someone to guide me, and I need to up my fitness. I cannot take the next steps on my own. There is ground within a reasonable distance of me, and in that place is someone who might be able to help.

But, he is different, and has a reputation for being difficult.

Mountain rescue is the progeny of tragedy.

As leisure time expanded in the early part of the twentieth century more people ventured outdoors and to ever more remote areas. Walking and climbing clubs sprang up, cavernous vicarages converted into hostels, public transport reached further away from home. With improvements to working hours, holidays and a plethora of social movements, for the ordinary person this was an age of exploration, of new experiences, of a growing sense of adventure. With it came mishaps and fatalities.

Lack of experience, inadequate clothing and equipment, and an almost universal ignorance of terrain, weather and their effects on the human body all led to an increase in such mishaps. The rise in requests for help and moments of tragedy brought the need for a co-ordinated, well-trained and equipped response to the attention of the authorities.

It was the police who were tasked with responding and organising search and rescue efforts, as they are today. As the seriousness and length of an incident unfolded police resources were augmented by walkers and climbers, local communities, farmers, members of the public. Images of the time show police in street uniform and civilians in basic hill gear struggling against the elements.

As it is today, the Peak District was popular with walkers and climbers who poured in on easy rail access from the surrounding towns and cities of the North and Midlands. The huge numbers inevitably leading to an increase in incidents.

The gloriously named Joint Stretcher Committee was an early response to the need for specialised equipment, resulting from a climbing accident at Laddow Rocks near Crowden in the late 1920s. The lack of suitable equipment necessitated the use of a field gate and rapidly adapted personal kit to extract the casualty over tortuous terrain. The climber would lose a limb; the need for specialist equipment to ease evacuation was identified as an issue in the rescue.

In the second half of the twentieth century, the Peak District saw some of the most traumatic and tragic incidents. An avalanche in the Chew Valley in 1963 claimed the life of two climbers caught in Wilderness Gully. The difficulty in raising the alarm and the subsequent delay and effectiveness of the response gave impetus for interested groups to come together to provide a better solution.

In 1964 three youths died while taking part in the Four Inns race during a winter storm. A team of four youths had found themselves forced into the narrow, steep-sided Alport Dale by the worsening weather that had descended on Bleaklow, a high barren landscape with little shelter. One managed to reach safety and raise the alarm, the others became trapped by the landscape. With inadequate clothing and insurmountable ground conditions the three succumbed and lost their lives. It took several days to find their bodies, the police calling on anyone capable of helping. Vast numbers arrived by train from the industrial heartlands. The search was hampered by heavy snowfall and freezing cold; photographs show police in greatcoats struggling through waist-high snow. The coroner noted the search was affected by a lack of formal organised response and effective communications. By the time of the inquest into the tragedy, changes were underway that would transform emergency response in the remote areas of Britain.

Today, forty-seven teams, some with additional cave rescue capabilities, cover the major outdoor and remote areas of England and Wales. Scotland and Northern Ireland also have mountain rescue services. Statistics from the national organising body, Mountain Rescue England and Wales, show that in 2021 the teams deployed to 2,881 incidents, dedicating almost 120,000 hours of volunteer time to help those in distress. Twenty per cent of call-outs were for missing people, the remainder responding to trauma. Each team spends tens of thousands of pounds annually, funded entirely by donation. Mountain rescue is respected around the world for its expertise in rescuing people. A far cry from the days of borrowing a farmer's five-bar gate.

Every team sits within the national body that forms the spine, providing contact with officialdom, sharing experience, skills, knowledge and equipment. Each individual team's own ecosystem – their DNA – has developed over decades by the nature of call-outs and the landscape in which they operate. There are ecosystems within ecosystems, like a Russian doll; the outer layer, the one holding them all, is the desire to help someone in distress.

Landscape and weather dictate the skills used, the equipment deployed, how an incident unfolds, revealing the unique identity of a team. A search in the Cairngorms in the depths of winter requires a vastly different skill set to a search in Wensleydale in summer. A team whose patch has a long crag – infested with countless climbing routes and close to the road – will out of necessity and practice be slickly proficient at picking up a mass of broken bones and scraped skin.

All teams will have their crag rats, rope knitters, human flies – liberating the crag-fast individual from peril, whose knees tremble, convinced this is the end, why did they ever start? There are the casualty carers, doctors, surgeons, paramedics, anaesthetists, lay people willing to put in the extra hours of learning to straighten limbs, stem the flow of blood, keep the heart pumping. The snatch squads, Lycra-clad, thin, young or old, sent racing up in ballet shoes so sparse in covering so plentiful of holes, they barely warrant the time to put them on, to intercept those in distress. The water babies, forever polishing their gear and living in hope. The comms, unintelligible words and concepts, the IT department – the next 'patch' will solve whatever issue is current. The drivers, smiling as they go off-road, or praying for a chance to use those blues and twos. The navigators with their dark arts of paper and compass, and never a secret told. The donkeys, the heavy-lifting gang, slogging up hills with kit that will almost certainly never be used, just in case. The stretcher carriers, the bag carriers, the ones who are there but people never see. The controllers, the search managers, the tea makers, the note takers, the backroom admin who dot the i's and cross the t's, so everything works. The supporters: tea, cake and rattle tins. Beware of a seemingly nice lady, proffering homemade Ferrero Rocher sprouts. Now you know. The dog handlers – 'grumpy bastards' – aloof loners trusting only their dog and the wind.

And, there are no heroes. Those who want to be, do not last. The badge collectors and the jacket wearers leave the real article to carry on with the work.

And there are grains of truth in all of that.

The notion of the lone dog section away from the rest of the team, searching out the secrets held within the landscape, listening to the story the wind tells, is undeniably romantic. I always think there is some truth in this when I view Caspar David Friedrich's painting *Wanderer Above the Sea of Fog*, not least in the mind of the handler. This romanticisation is part mindset, part necessity. The team facing the landscape as one, away from the surrounding world, searching out the lie of the land, leaning into the oncoming wind to hear what secrets it tells. The loneliness of a dog search team.

The attraction for me lies in the two non-human components. A landscape that is truthful, handing freedom to humans if respected, but punishment if treated foolishly. And a dog who trusts, once it has selected and trained the right human. Scout trusts me completely. We are one, seeking out the anomaly. Our world is a patch of ground, a mountain, a hillside. Standing ready to step into the search we are at the mercy of my confidence. I must not let him down.

Only a handler can say what their dog is best placed to do. A search manager takes note of the handler's advice, marshalling his resources to keep their scent away from the dog team, giving them a clean area, uncontaminated by search sections. Dogs are better suited to some terrains and times of day than humans; a boulder field at night is no fun for a tall unstable biped, great fun for a lively quadruped. Bramble-covered waste ground is no fun for soft paws and a sensitive nose, but no issue for heavy boots. A woodland is simpler to search by a nose, a football field by a pair of eyes. Scout loves boulder fields but is not a fan of brambles.

The unique skill of a dog team makes them a national asset – they can be asked to operate anywhere in the country. This increases the number of call-outs attended, making the dog and handler the busiest team members. A search can last a few minutes, the person found before boots and paws have hit the ground. Or hours, days, even weeks, with dozens of dog teams arriving from far afield.

For me and Scout, this is yet to be. We still have far to travel.

A handler's role is to ensure an area is searched with a high degree of certainty. The missing person is either located, or not there at the time of the search – hence *clearing the area*. Place a dog's nose in a scent cone and it will work its way to the source. Ensuring the nose is in the right place is my job.

It has been a long time since I have trained with a local handler. There is only one handler in the previous group who I feel could and would help, but they regularly work away. I need consistency for the next stages of training. Working on my own these last twelve months have been good, but I do not possess the knowledge to take us further.

There is a group of handlers in the North. They're seen as mavericks because of their different approach, plain speaking and resistance to suffering fools. I have watched them on national courses, listened to their discussions and banter, noticed that handlers and bodies take note, found what they say, and do, matches. If I find a person saying one thing but doing another, I disengage. Permanently. Trust is my primary touchstone. I make the call.

It's the first conversation I have had with Steve, and I'm apprehensive. I tell him what my training needs are: to learn how to search an area efficiently. He says he's heard and seen what's happened in the last eighteen months; he doesn't pass comment. I ask if he can help me. Immediately he says yes, but I hear caution in his voice. For a long time, I hold the phone staring blankly out of the window.

I hope I have found my mentor to guide me. After months of being in the wilderness my spirit is high, I can see all is possible. He gives me instructions to meet the coming Sunday. I'm to wait with Scout and my hill kit by a locked gate.

. . .

It's a long drive over Saddleworth Moor. The bleak landscape, even in summer, has rugged beauty, but a sinister brooding keeps a low murmur. Evil lingers on the lonely highway. Children, drawn into the wilderness, tortured, murdered, dumped in peaty graves, some never to be found. Their screams held in the wind.

It will be our training ground for operational assessment, the closest I have to the testing areas in Wales and Cumbria. It is shaped like a huge bowl, the base filled with water, the sides rising sharply through boulder fields and gritstone crags, and beyond the rim, nothingness that goes on to the horizon. It is a harsh place, difficult to work, studded with tussocky grass hiding leg-breaking holes saturated with fetid water and peat. The smell of rotting life smears shins and hands, fingertips worn raw by grit-laden peat as hands seek to break a fall, the rank blood of the moor seeping into skin through waterlogged wool and leather. Many handlers fear this place: the terrain, the weather, the demands on fitness, the courage needed to dance across boulders and tiptoe the face of crags.

We meet by the gate, pleasantly pass the time. I'm told to leave my van, to walk, while others drive. Trust yet to be established. I acquiesce, grab my pack. With Scout on his lead, we step on to Chew Road.

The Office is a group of indistinct rocks on a small knoll. Wedged into cracks are bits of tat – old slings, frayed lengths of rope, a figure of eight on a bight – harsh weather having gnawed away their colour. Errant dogs are attached, the scrappers and unknowns. Scout sits, tethered, watching dogs play a few feet away, investigating wildlife calling cards.

I wait, unsure of the etiquette. Steve, my mentor (prospective), asks where we are in our training. I hesitate, not knowing how much he is aware of. I plunge, speaking plainly, and honestly, keeping to my responsibility. I don't want to get in the middle of factions or be denigrating anyone. I keep to what we can do, what we can't, what I think I know and don't. My two major issues are ranging – Scout staying too close, making me cover more of the ground which takes longer. And directional control – moving Scout around by command – is poor verging on non-existent. I don't give the answers I think they want. It's a short conversation.

In front of the Office is a flat expanse of moor, tussocks of grass every-where, islands of rock, a deep channel running top to bottom. There are three bodies, location known to me. It's my job to get Scout into the scent cone for a strike on each. Behind me handlers have fallen quiet, eyes on me stepping on to the moor, the space expanding to infinity, the loneliest place on earth.

I slip Scout's lead, stroke his ears, feel the wind. It's moving top to bottom. We begin at the bottom to work into it. I'm tense and rigid. Scout sets off and begins asking for his toy. My anger wells up. I try and push him out with different inflections of my voice, light, growling. He keeps up the barking, spinning wildly, bouncing up and down, each landing punctuated with a bark. The wind throws arrows of failure into my body, seeking out the tenderest conditioning of a childhood. *Why now, Scout?* It's worse than ever. I'm at the point of walking away and never returning.

Over the radio Steve tells me to stop, give Scout some love and calm things down. I do. Scout does. We begin again having not moved from our starting point in the last ten minutes. It's the same. More suggestions float out of the radio. I try. I really try. *Why is he doing this?* After ten more minutes we've only moved forwards because I have, and no body has been found.

We stop again and calm things down. I feel alone. Between me and the Office a desert has appeared. A few minutes of rest, more time ticking away, more time spent stationary while handlers look on. I can feel every bone and muscle in my neck pulling tight. We move off again. Still the same. Scout doesn't want to understand. I'm struggling to get words out, the world has shrunk to the metre of ground we inhabit, the sound of Scout fills the unending moor. The mist descends.

I'm holding Scout's head; it's clamped between my hands. Words are screaming out of my mouth telling him to go and find the body, our lips so close I see the white flecks of my spittle spattering his nose. His eyes ever widening showing surprise, the words punched in bold with big fat periods: 'FIND. HIM. OUT.'

There is no sound, the mist evaporates, my hands relax. Scout drops to the ground, ears back, eyes searching mine. Sweat dripping down my back, breath labouring, lungs wailing, brain whirling.

In a low voice I say, 'find him out.' He leaves, ranging out well. My heavy legs drag me after him, depression pressing down on each shoulder saying *I'm no good*. Scout cuts across the wind; his nose snapping right, he strikes and is out of my sight. I hear the bark, see him heading back to me, excitement and willingness to please beaming from his face. He speaks and springs back to the body. When I reach him, the toy sails high and I'm over the top with praise, emotionally wrecked, wracked with guilt. Scout happily plays with the body, the immediate past gone. Now is now. I'm not here with him, I'm back there when I think I saw in his eyes the fear I had put there.

We move off for the second body; the barking and dancing resume. I shout, 'find him out.' He half complies, half hesitates, unsure what comes next. I say it again, go quiet, my mind disengaging to freewheel through what future we have. The second body is found, Scout indicating perfectly.

I'm pulled back to the Office. With a body still to find I know this is a fail. At the Office handlers and bodies move away. Only the two senior handlers stay; I know this is the end.

Steve, the mentor (prospective), steps up to me as I tie Scout to some tat.

'Right. The first thing. We do not use aggression in any form with our dogs. A strong word yes, but not fear. The dog does not deserve that, it serves no purpose. We use rewards here. It is not the dog's fault they are not doing what we want. It is ours.'

'I'm sorry. That's never happened before.'

'We are guessing things you have been taught, things you have seen, have led you down that path. It is just wrong.'

'I just got so frustrated.'

'Dog training is ninety per cent frustration. So, get used to it. Now that we have observed what you and Scout can do, we can begin to train you properly, as a proper dog team. Scout has a good indication, clearly knows the game, so what you have done together on your own is good. The essentials are there. You have had to train on your own a lot, have you not?'

'Yes, it was the only way.'

'Well, you have done a good job, and you were right to come to us. If that is what you still want.'

There's no nastiness, no shouting at me to fuck off.

'Yes. It is what I want. I would be very grateful.'

'Good. We will set another area up and this time work on getting Scout to move off without all that palaver. It may be that we will not achieve that, it seems pretty ingrained. We have seen lots of dogs that have trained as you were taught at the beginning. The constant repetition of the same sequence imprints it on the dog's mind and if they do not move on soon the dog becomes addicted. That is not your fault, you followed what others told you to do. You are with us now and we have a different approach to training. What we do is all our responsibility, but especially yours with Scout. We are here to help and guide each other.'

I relax on to the rock by Scout, watch the other dogs play, pop a treat into his mouth, ruffle his coat. He looks at me, holding me. 'I'm sorry,' I tell him. He looks, then he eyes my treat pocket.

We have found our home.

•   •   •

The waters in Chew Reservoir, once England's highest reservoir until they built another somewhere else, somewhere higher, sits at the head of the steep-sided Chew Valley. Chew Brook, its flow across the moor from Black Chew Head interrupted by the man-made lake, continues out of the dam, slides underneath Chew Road, splitting the valley in two as it slips over gritstone to the valley below. Other brooks tumble down other valleys; only Chew Brook has a companion alongside, Chew Road.

The palette of the valley is brown. And black. Most of the year. The silver-black thread of water runs down its spine. The land is a contradiction of drab and boring, ominous and unsettling, verdant and glorious. The colours are seasonal: dull yellows, browns and black in the depths of the long winters. Luscious greens burst forth after rain in spring. Autumn brings reds and golds as the valley claws at the sun. In summer the bracken is waist high, in places head high; it is difficult to move through the tangle of stalks and hothouse microclimate within. Pink heather from long-abandoned grouse shoots splatters the hillside; the carefree descendants complain at errant humans from beneath the rampant thick cover. Both plants have bolted through lack of sheep and burn, the woody heather scratching legs, polishing boots and undoing laces. The vibrant bracken lassoing legs. The ground has long since receded, making it impossible to see feet firmly planted.

Tussocky grass, baby's heads in these parts, feigns benign cover across the open moor, invading the spaces between bracken, heather and gritstone. It is neither short nor tall, reaching knee high at best, forming random patterns of rounded clumps rooted in wet peaty soil, the structure highly unstable though curiously firmly anchored. Between each head and its neighbour is a dead space of generally firm ground, the width of a single boot, allowing the experienced to cross the moor using the labyrinth hidden from sight by the grass sprouting out of the top of the baby's heads.

There is a catch. Sometimes the boot rests not on firm ground but is enveloped by slimy sludgy pools of stagnant water that fills boots with a putrid stench, socks absorbing the cold soup of rotting debris and creatures best not thought about. This is not the worst of it.

Sometimes there is no terra firma. The boot along with foot plunging to the centre of the earth, the sound of water and saturated peat sucking like a blocked drain. All too late for the inexperienced, the momentum drives the foot deeper while the body continues forwards, the dry foot on firm ground, the groin, hamstring, tendon and knee straining, the weight of the pack taking the body beyond its centre of gravity, until *crack*. The tibia snaps, or a hamstring, or knee, maybe a forearm or shoulder thrust out to break the fall to no avail. Spectacles, if worn, never to be found. The human felled.

Days of saturating rain engorge peat, the well-watered land hiding a morass of bog unable to hold the weight of a human. The hapless have to be pulled free, two feet minus boots and socks.

Handlers not versed in the art of moorland walking spend a lot of time falling over, expending precious energy trying to keep feet dry, to look competent. The whole pantomime ending with a hand clutching hopelessly at razor-sharp grass and vanishing dignity.

Boulders lie at the foot of the crag, line the banks of Chew Brook, gather like old women in social groups on the moor. In summer when the bracken is high the boulders play hide and seek. Scent loves this game, loves their nooks and crannies, the warm rock to settle by, drawing dogs into the jumble, the handler following, hoping each footstep reaches a solid something rather than airy nothing.

The sides of the valley are very steep, winnowing out the unfit. Battling through bracken and heather while ascending is wearing on mind and body. Add in keeping an eye on a dog, ensuring ground is covered, dancing over boulders, skipping precarious ground, and it's exhausting. It isn't easy for the dogs either. Small breeds disappear before human eye, worn out by the constant battle with the environment. Big breeds find bog trotting and rock hopping hard going and display a tendency for a renegotiation of working conditions.

The final assessment of a search dog team takes place in the harshest of conditions and terrain. Hence why I, acting as a body in 2015, was lying on a Welsh mountain in winter, in a gully, by the side of a raging torrent, high up on a series of ledges backed by towering cliffs. It was icily cold. It had rained all day, and the day before that, and the day before that one. Water poured down the mountain, the sound obliterating any thought as it crashed to the valley floor. The ground was a sodden mush that skidded boots across the hillside, the rock greasy and petulant. The exposure was relentless. The potential for serious injury ever-present. The conditions perfect. I was happily waiting to be found by a dog team on their first area of their first assessment. Comfortable, warm in my bivvy, a view through sheets of rain at what I knew to be a glorious Welsh valley.

A barking dog brought the sight of a human shakily crabbing on all fours across the rock, repeating the mantra that this was too dangerous, that they should not have to do this, home was nothing like this. The dog, having crossed the stream, wagged its tail. 'You must move,' the human screamed. I reassured them I was fine, offered them a brew. Shaking their head they precariously descended to the valley floor, dog skipping ahead with joy, reached their car, drove away, career as a search dog team over before it had begun.

They say make it in Chew Valley and a dog team can make it anywhere.

A handler tells me when they began training in Chew Valley, they made rapid progress and knew they were a better team because of the people there. It is gratifying to hear I've made a good choice. The support is excellent, open and honest from the beginning, everyone wanting each dog team to do well.

Our progress is steady, each session building upon the previous. There's homework, techniques to be tried or mastered. Nothing is taken for granted. Just because one dog team is successful with a way of working does not mean all dogs must follow; this methodology dissipates much of the frustration that precipitated our journey into the wilderness. Scout likes it too. No longer tethered, he joins in play with the other dogs. Both of us are enjoying ourselves; that romantic image of dog and man alone against the elements is coalescing into reality.

Scout still has the remnants of his bark and dance routine at the beginning of a search, but we've incorporated it into his warm-up, letting him get the excitement out of his system, warming his joints and muscles for the work ahead. He's ranging well, allowing me time to pay more attention to the land still needing to be covered. With larger areas we have small breaks, a few minutes every half hour, to relax mind and body, take on sustenance, review progress, make any radio calls. I spend the occasional long night staring at the ceiling trying to work out how to achieve a desired behaviour from Scout.

We cover larger areas now, Steve setting ever more intricate challenges. I've realised that Scout likes to be left alone to work the scent without a flow of instructions from me. I restrict interruptions with a few words of direction and support. It's the opposite of how Steve works – his voice booms around the valley, a stream of encouragement radiating out. He transfers this to the radio when Scout and I are working, his voice pouring out of the speaker with perfectly good advice, often not wanted at that exact moment. As the weeks have gone on, I've become less and less appreciative to hear the radio spring into life and his dulcet Yorkshire tones rattle across the moor. It comes to a head as I'm crossing tussocky ground trying to keep up with Scout. The radio buzzes into life. Now, as I write, I cannot remember what Steve said, all I retain is the feeling of guilt when I exploded and told this man who had gone out of his way to help me, to shut up. In disgust at myself I switch the radio off, spending the rest of the exercise burnishing my selfishness. The walk back to the Office is a torment. The very least I owe is an apology.

'I'm sorry,' I say. 'I think we work better quietly. I should have said.'

'No, you were quite correct,' Steve grins. 'Now we know talking does not help we will keep quiet and debrief back at the Office. It's time we learned how to handle you.'

A handler prods his finger in my side and tells me I'm a big baby.

As summer rolls in, Alison and I take the dogs up to Scotland. We've spent the last ten years working our way up the north-west coast, starting in Ardnamurchan, taking in the islands, staying in remote cottages to get access to sea and mountain top. This will be Scout's first time scaling a Munro. We have a stalkers' cottage nestled at the foot of Glas Bheinn. Our days are gentle: a stroll into the village, the dogs swimming in the sea loch, a run through a pine forest, the tracks deserted. Our Munro expedition takes us from Coulags along the course of the Fionn-abhainn. After a rest at the bothy, we swing left to follow Allt Mnatha Luadhadair to the bealach, then turn right up to the 933-metre summit of Maol Chean-dearg, its slopes covered in Torridon stone and sharp quartz. It's a wonderful walk, the walk-in one of the best approaches to any mountain.

The clear stream flows hard. Even with the hot days of late, there are a few pools that Scout and Olly take advantage of while Monty roots around the path. It's after the bothy that we notice Monty is missing. After an hour of calling there is no sight of him; Alison is distraught. I go back to where we last saw him, my search training taking me to the 'place last seen'. He isn't there. I call for an hour. Monty appears high above me, trying to work out how much trouble he is in. He spends the rest of the walk on the lead with Alison. At the summit we sit and take in the view over Applecross to the Isle of Skye and the Cuillins. Our return takes longer, tired legs on our biggest day out.

At two-and-a-bit years old, Scout is almost fully grown and filling his muscles with strength and energy. More days like this will be good for both our fitness levels. I think there is a possibility that we could go for assessment in November – five search areas over three days – a big call on energy and strength. We'll need some cardio work. If there is one thing that holds me up it's my breathing. It doesn't stop me, but I have a sense that it could be a lot better.

A search is not guesswork. Profiles of missing people are used to inform search managers of likely behaviour and support decisions of where to look, and what resources to deploy.

A seasoned walker's failure to return home, the weather rapidly deteriorating, presents a likelihood that they may have found shelter, bunkered down behind a wall, managed to get into a valley. If they are injured, they will hopefully reach protection; if not, they may lie unconscious somewhere, anywhere. The inexperienced walker, in the belief that safety is just around the corner, over the next hill, may keep moving, even moving in and out of search areas, making them harder to locate. Teams will seal off land with human barriers along possible escape routes to capture the hapless wanderer.

Children – and adults with dementia – often succumb to confusion and tiredness as they seek their way out. They take cover in buildings, beneath a hedge, in a bracken-laden hollow, sometimes burrowing deep into seemingly inaccessible places.

People wanting to end their life will often choose a spot that has meaning for the final moment.

Climbers are generally found at the foot of the crag or dangling halfway up; mountain bikers around the biggest tree or boulder; scantily clad fell runners rarely go missing. Tourists move only short distances from the car park.

A search is the elimination of probability. The most effective tools a search manager has are experience and a wet black nose.

Summer is hot and dry. There have been several moorland fires, the land loaded with tinder-dry heather, the proverbial barbecue tray found at the seat of the conflagration. Blue smoke drifts into the towns and cities, the acrid tang choking throats and stinging eyes. It's impossible to work or train in these conditions. When the land has cooled, the vast swathes of charred peat and heather make for a quick and easy passage across the moor.

The heat has brought thousands of people into the hills to escape the concrete and brick canyons of the towns and cities, ramping up the team's workload. Lost walkers, broken bones, traumatised mountain bikers, dehydrated runners – all are suffering. I do a lot of stretcher carries, picking up my old role as one of the donkeys. It isn't pleasant, sweat pouring down on to hands that are struggling to keep a grip on hot metal frames. Most people are relieved to see us; only occasionally do we arrive to find we may not be so welcome. It's where diplomacy comes in handy, a little firmness with a casualty who is less in control of their emotions than they would perhaps like.

Strong-minded little old ladies are often the most troublesome. Hiking with friends, the roll of a boot leading to a broken ankle. When we arrive, the 'friends' are sat chatting, eating lunch, draining flasks of coffee. The casualty a little way off sulkily berating her friends for calling out mountain rescue. The presence of a road just a few hundred metres across a stream and in sight – with spectacles – is ample proof that her son-in-law could be summoned irrespective of whether he was at work or not. The white and pink fleshy bone sticking out nothing more than a scratch that the first aid kit in the Quality Street tin at home would sort out in a jiffy. She is sorry for all the trouble and inconvenience, it was their fault – the 'friends' – who had gone soft after they'd had double glazing fitted. We needn't bother. We could go home. A few firm words from the biggest team member, and, reluctantly, the feisty lady let herself be rescued. As we stretchered past her friends, the painkilling Entonox being consumed with gusto, they waved bye-bye to her boozy smile.

We get calls to find dementia patients who have escaped from their care home, the doors and windows open for cool air. Many are trying to reach a place of meaning, a connection from long ago. They can be gone for several days, surviving without food and water until found in some unfathomable place.

As days increase for someone missing, a search expands pulling more teams in from across the country. An experienced seventy-year-old walker missing in North Yorkshire is found alive after three days – one hundred mountain rescue team members and thirteen search dogs from across the North of England helped find them. Each rescuer stepping away from their daily life of home and work to help a stranger.

The recurring mishaps and serious errors in judgement, some fatal, bring condemnation across social media from keyboard warriors. Teams never comment. It isn't the rescuer's job to criticise. 'There but for the grace go I', a well-placed maxim.

Days pass punctuated with spikes of activity. Scout helps research my latest guidebook in the South Pennines. It's an area that is new to us, full of interesting communities, a mix of farming and old industry, wool and cotton still present after the work has long ceased. He makes another appearance at Sheffield train station, his fan base surrounding him to cover him with kisses, drop a few pounds in the team's collection bucket, even the odd celebrity posing with him.

In the dog days of summer, we are training on Bodmin Moor, a lunar landscape of yellow plains and grey granite. There is no shade. There are no trees. The sun pulls moisture from the surface leaving humans dry. It could not be more different from the wet peat bogs of the Chew Valley, yet both landscapes are as dangerous to unwary humans.

I feel we are ready for our next test. I've been extending Scout's working time and stamina to enable us to work comfortably for longer. We need to show we can work for sixty minutes efficiently and skilfully. Passing the next stage will place us in striking distance of the final assessment and ready in time for the winter crop of lost and injured. I grab five minutes with the instructor to discuss a test. They'll need to see us first.

The second day is very hot. I'm working an area with the Second Man, to simulate working together which is common on large and complicated searches. We are at a trig pillar looking down at the plain we have to search. To the right and ahead is grass, some sheep in a corner. To the left is the granite ridge we stand on running out to the bulge of a tor. Below is a boulder field, almost hidden by bracken. Far below, behind us, the Office.

I'm carrying as much water as I can, and already sweating. It's quickly apparent we are working an environment we've never experienced. There is no wind, just uniform heavy air that has no movement, a blanket of heat that blinds the scent, the landscape shimmering in thick transparent waves. We work small areas to pick up scent, but Scout is soon looking for shade and guzzling down water. We reduce working time to twenty minutes, then ten, and rest. I let Scout cover the land how he wants, keeping a close eye for any signs of heat exhaustion. We find the bodies, sweating away under camouflage tarps. I don't encourage any play reward, and Scout doesn't want it, he slips under a rock letting the cooler earth refresh his torso. The bodies are relieved at being out of their sauna, and more relieved they don't have to jump up and down. They take on water. We have just the granite tor to clear, but I've lost any thoughts of the test. At the tor it's clear Scout is not happy, moving from shade to shade, his pink tongue lolling far out of the side of his mouth, his chest heaving, his eyes pleading for an end to the torment. We rest in shade for twenty minutes, drink water, pour the final drops along his back. We begin again and find the body, then head straight down to the river. Scout launches himself in, luxuriating in the coldness wrapping around his body as he swims in a large circle, happy. I dangle my feet in and think about the exercise. I've learned an important lesson. We need to manage our resources, pay attention to conditions. Until now, focus has been on bad weather training, but this benign-looking landscape has been our most brutal experience. It has taken its toll on me as well. Along with the sweat and dehydration, I've been uneasy with my breathing, the heat torching my lungs, reducing their capacity to a pant.

We are not ready for the test.

I can feel both of us teeming into one mould, melding together, our bond strong. More and more I'm leaving Scout to his own devices in a search, just dropping the occasional direction to look here or there. It feels wonderful. Is wonderful. The larger training areas give us much more time together and more space for Scout to range. We're becoming like a long-time married couple communicating without words, knowing what each will do before it happens. I've taken to choosing vantage points to watch him work the land-scape and give me a moment to rest.

With the heat turning high moors into crucibles, we've taken to the cool of a forest evening for training. It's an old royal hunting forest surrounding a large chase and impressive crags. There's ancient woodland of oak and beech, stands of commercial pine, some beautiful Scots pine. Dotted within are pockets of pasture and long-forgotten platforms where charcoal burners spent long days and nights tending a burn. The forest teems with wildlife. Owls and raptors are plentiful, the sound of cuckoo and woodpecker piercing the quiet, deer gather in secluded valleys, badgers build extensive setts away from human form. There is a network of tracks and a web of foot-paths and hidden trails that run like roots of the trees. Several streams and a plunge pool bring coolness. It is well frequented by local people – walkers, dogs, horse riders, mountain bikers – most staying on the tracks. It's a regular call-out for the team, mountain bikers hitting immovable objects, always the same ones, decelerating instantly, their bodies absorbing the trauma of impact, rupturing kidneys and spleens, breaking necks and backs.

Our training is going well and I'm wanting to work on the finer points of air scenting: seeing how environmental elements affect how human molecules act, and how Scout and I respond. Annette and Diane have joined Paul to increase our search times and create different scenarios within one training session. I've asked them to hide in specific locations early in the evening to allow their scent pools to build. I'm interested to see what happens when the day begins to cool and thermal currents reverse, pulling scent down to the valley bottom.

Annette is under brambles in the ancient part of the wood. We'd recently had a multi-team search for a dementia patient who had absconded from his care home. He'd been missing two days, the search area covering many square miles. He'd been found alive huddled deep in brambles – in an area that had already been searched by a human foot section surmising no one could enter the spiky thorns – by a search dog walking high above in the early morning, the sun lifting the scent into the path of the dog. He was 200 metres from the care home.

Diane is hiding under a bush on the blind side of a wall. It will be interesting to see how Scout responds. I wonder if we need to be a certain distance away from the wall to detect a scent dump flowing over it from Diane.

Paul is hiding in an unknown location. I've given him general directions: left at the first track junction, walk one hundred metres, walk into the trees on the right for one hundred metres. I don't want to know his exact position; I want Scout to work for it.

It's a beautiful evening, sunbeams through the trees, the golden shafts alive with motes of the forest. A light breeze drifts from high ground as I had expected, showing my learning is leading to understanding. I'm taking Scout on a long arc so we can approach Paul from downwind, and I can watch and learn what the scent is doing and how Scout responds. He's relaxed, freewheeling down the track in low gear, investigating the dog-world's social media posts. I like how he flicks through the comments, his mind ticking over as he scrolls, his tongue quivering at a bush, a gate post. Rex was here, and Millie, but who is that? Scout posts a comment: 'Scout was here.' I let him unwind his mind; soon enough he will be engaging with my world, a little time with his own friends won't hurt.

I've added a bell to the red light on his working coat. Now he is ranging far he's often out of sight; the bell tells me he is moving and in what area. When it goes quiet, he'll be checking out a scent dump or will have found a body. Then I'll hear the chime drifting towards me.

When he's finished with his social media posts I slip his coat on and give him a big hug, tell him how much I love him. I get a sideways glance, his eyes going white, the tan brow dancing above. I know he thinks this is silly, but I cherish these moments. 'Find him out.' Off he goes.

The ground is dry, the early sounds of autumn crunching under his paws sending blackbirds into the forest canopy, darkening in the fading light, the day just a few metres high. We have the breeze at our back to see how Scout responds as we pass Annette. She is a superb dogsbody, almost impossible to see even when close, and like Paul, Annette and Scout love each other and their play time. Diane is new; they've both got to get used to each other, learn the ways, and that's good because Scout will rarely know the people he is sent to find.

I'm zigzagging through a strip of trees to ensure I cross Annette's scent cone. Scout's nose snaps back into the drifting breeze and begins drilling the air a metre above the ground, working to a patch of bramble, fallen trees, mounds of rotting wood. He tries to find a way in, the thorns making him tentative; his desire to find keeps him probing. I stand downwind and encourage him to encircle the clump. He sticks his nose into a tiny void in the nest, then a little further, then his head disappears. The tail begins wagging happiness. He steps back, examines the spot, looks at me, barks. 'Show me.' The nose points at the black hole; he does not attempt to re-enter. He isn't stupid. It takes a while for my eyes to grow accustomed to the darkness, arranging light and shade into order; a camouflage tarp slowly materialises. It's Annette. It's a great hide and a super find. The scent cone has crept through the undergrowth snagging on branches and leaf, trailing long wisps on the day's settling breath.

We move on. Diane is not far away, behind a wall on our right. Scout ambles along as I direct him left and right of the dusty path, the wind still behind us. At Diane's spot he continues as if nothing has happened, until he gets to the corner of the wall when his nose snaps back and he begins following the wall back to a spot where he concentrates hard on the ground, then above, then a little away from the wall, scribing a cube in the space. He hasn't looked at me, kept his nose sampling, sharp snorts lifting leaf off the ground. Back to the wall, tracing the joints, steps back and looks at it. He knows there is human scent. It could be a scent dump from earlier in the day, a person leaning on the wall to look at the lush green pasture beyond. 'Find him out.' He barks. I help him out, tap the top of the wall. I still don't know whether Diane is here, but scent is. Another tap on the wall. 'Find him out.' He jumps on top, head looking down the other side. Bark. 'Good boy!' There is Diane, close into the wall, like someone finding protection from the weather. It's a good find. One he had to think through, with a little help. This isn't a problem – we work as a team; the more we experience different scenarios the more we will instinctively understand what to do.

We follow thin trails down the valley, human or animal, probably both.

The air is dense around my legs, degrees lighter round my head, a miasma rising and falling with the thermal exchange of the closing day. Scout, free of his working coat, explores streams, takes on water, happy and relaxed.

At the bottom of the forest, we reset. The coat on, a kiss and a hug, that teenager's scowl, then the command. We work into the scent being pulled down to us. All the people who have walked the dog, all the mountain bikers, the kids who've been making dens, the deer stepping back into trees, the rabbit held in the buzzard's claw, they are all here, molecules of life drifting into Scout's nose.

I reckon less than half an hour before we reach Paul. But we don't.

When we get to the position I expect Paul to be, Scout passes by. I've been moving him from one side of the track to the other, looking for the scent cone; I would have guaranteed that Scout would have a strike, we are after all moving into the breeze. I direct Scout to the location; he finds nothing. We do a full 360-degree pass. Nothing. Paul is not here and hasn't been. My directions must have been unclear; maybe Paul has gone on the opposite side of the track. We go back to our set-up point and reset. It's hard work on the forest floor in this section. The aftermath of commercial pine logging has left the floor strewn with brash and trunks, everything barring a few green spaces covered in bramble. I move from one green patch to the next, stumbling through a tangle of thorns, my hands full of tiny spikes, the palms pricking with red blood.

After thirty minutes Scout lifts his head and pecks the air; his shape dissolves into the foliage, his bell sparkling in the falling dusk. Scout appears to tell me, does his little dance and only stops barking when I tell him to show me. He's quickly off; I'm having trouble keeping up, my clumsy legs getting tied up in strong briars. He comes back several times, his frustration louder each time. When finally I reach the spot there is nothing. He's stood in a small clearing, tale swishing like mad, eyes firmly on the pocket for his toy. Beyond is a small stream and beyond that head-high bracken. Peeking above the bracken the roots of a large fallen tree and beyond that the darkness of the forest. By Scout is a fallen Scots pine, others towering above encircle it like mourners. The floor is soft pine needles. I listen. The only sound is birds beginning to settle down for the night. There is no human sound. 'Show me.' Scout raises his eyebrows, eyes open wide, an aggressive bark splits the silence. I must be useless if I cannot see the body. After ten minutes I figure someone must have been here in the day, a picnic spot maybe, sat on the fallen tree, communed with nature. The breeze now flowing across the brook must have carried the scent to Scout's nose. I tell him to get on with the search and walk away. He stands his ground, barking, pounding the pine needles until they float all around him. He stands on the fallen tree in protest. He is really mad. I look up, half expecting to see the soles of someone's shoes. No human is quietly swaying in the trees. Maybe he wants a drink. At the stream he's manic. I've had enough, I thought we had got past all this. I walk away forcing him to follow me. Paul is not here. We've wasted another thirty minutes. Scout complains bitterly all the way back to the track.

I radio Paul who explains the route he has taken. He is at the next junction up. It's my poor directions. But what worries me most is Scout's behaviour. The shadow of the early days rears its head. What if scent dumps are so confusing to him that he cannot tell the difference from a body?

From Paul's junction I step across a small stream and take a cycle track down through old woodland to begin once again working into the breeze. Scout turns sharp into a stream; I let him run so he can clear his senses and have a drink; he's soon absorbed into the gloom. I follow the track almost to the beginning when I see bracken on my left swaying back and forth, getting closer to me, and a bell chiming. Scout emerges, his head poking out of the jungle. A double take has me located – eyes meet, he bounds forwards, barks, spins around, disappears back down the portal. I follow, my bulk pressing hard against the high bracken, my feet out of sight; I can only see green, the only direction I have is Scout's bell. Hot and sweaty, I reach a huge root ball from an upturned tree, grey with age, the roots poking above the bracken. But no Scout. And no tinkling bell. I call him. His head peeks, peek-a-boo, around the grey mass, his fur covered in torn green vegetation. Another bark and another drift of eyes. As I step forwards a human foot appears by Scout's leg, then the rest of Paul, snug against the tree roots. Scout sits upright, proud, his tail sweeping dust into the dying sunbeams. It's a cracking find.

'This is a great spot,' I tell Paul, as he pulls and tugs the toy with Scout. He says he was beginning to worry he had got the wrong place especially when he saw us half an hour ago. No, this is a good spot I say. It's well hidden, even has some water that I think Scout used to track you on.

Something isn't right. I go back through the evening until the penny drops.

'What do you mean half an hour ago, Paul?'

'You were just there', he says, pointing down to the stream. 'Seemed to be for ages, I could definitely hear Scout.'

As I move below Paul, I come to the stream Scout tracked in on. Across the water a pretty little open piece of ground, in the centre a fallen Scots pine resting on a bed of needles, looking down on it a congregation of tall

Scots pine forms a forest arboretum. It's the spot where Scout took me to earlier. Where he was so insistent he had found Paul. As now, the breeze and the water were drifting Paul's scent across the stream and dumping it in this gathering of pine. If I had worked Scout across the water, we would have found Paul half an hour earlier. I just wasn't experienced enough to work it out.

I talk it through with Steve later, laying out every single detail: wind direction, temperature, water, previous finds. He knows exactly what has happened, it's as I describe. I need to pay more attention to what Scout is saying to me. When Scout first came back and did his little dance and bark, not leaving, he was telling me he'd found something – there wasn't a body, but I needed to come and have a look. Operationally, it could have been some clothing discarded by someone experiencing hypothermia, that sort of thing. Or as this evening, the casualty close by. I now have two indications from Scout: one he's found a human, the second he's found something I need to investigate. The other thing I need to learn, that is what most handlers have to learn, is that Scout knows much more than me, always will. So, trust your dog.

Autumn finds us in the golden warmth of the Chew Valley clearing an area of steep land plunging down from the craggy fringe to the knife edge, cut through hundreds of millions of years by Chew Brook. It is a layer cake of time. Of Kinder Grit pushing out between wilderness and the sky. Grains of sand and quartz atop the other for too long to fathom, pressed together, their own weight squeezing forgotten breezes out of long horizons along the valley, blackened in the blink of geological time, the waters cutting deeper as the crags rise higher. Of a tumble of boulders calved from the face over those millions of years, quarried by patient water and, later, impatient hands frozen red and raw from the cold of steel, wind and ice wanting only to be somewhere warm away from this hell. Within the silt, the land slopes through shale and thin layers of coal, through endless time. Self-seeding holds thin soil for rough edgeland plants to colonise, the heather now free of human hands. A flat round disc of land sits on one side of a fall line, facing the sky, offering respite to ankles tentatively picking their way across the slope. The flatness falls away sharply, running out like a tide to the lower boulder field stretched along the shallow banks of the brook. These boulders are the entry way to the crags high above; all life must dance over this threshold, and before that the brook with its tumbling silver-black water stained with peat, the smoothed rock slick and greasy to human foot.

We have progressed from playing in the park with children running around, to chasing screaming adults across the moor, to me taking Scout to the body. Now, we know nothing. Not how many bodies, nor where they are, indeed if there are any at all. Our task is to clear the area methodically: if a body is there, we will find it; if it is not, we will say with confidence the area is clear. We are with the big dogs now.

Soon, Scout will be three. Hard work has filled out his body with lean strong muscle. The thing we both need is stamina to work a full day on the hill. We've already completed one exercise area this morning, not steep, but difficult. I worry that a second area so soon after will be too much. I keep this to myself and try to exude nonchalant confidence, flicking the demon off my shoulder.

I outline my search plan to the instructors who will be watching. A firm northerly is rising steadily up the valley. We will begin on the southern boundary, weaving west up the slopes to the crag. It's the most efficient way, the wind driving scent straight into Scout's nose for the easy strike. The clock starts when we set foot on the bridge crossing Chew Brook.

Scout leads me up Chew Road, nipping into a ditch to take in some cool water while I study the idiosyncrasies of the landscape: the folds, dips, clumps of vegetation, rocks, noting unusual features to use as markers when we are moving through the area. As I work, I know perspective and time will expand and contract, the land shape-shifting, what was small looming large, near becoming far away. What was visible, as the instructor's finger traced the boundary of the search area, will become invisible. Being inside the landscape is very different to being outside looking in.

Scout is eager to get on, pulling the lead hard, the smell of water putting his senses into high gear – maybe he wants a drink. As soon as I slip him off, he scoots across the bridge and sharp left, paws scraping clouds of dust from the dry ground, down to the brook. I figure a drink, clearing his olfactory chambers after the morning search. He's quick – back before I am halfway across – and looks odd, crouching, his eyes ablaze. I say nothing. Probably a new twist in his start procedure. He lunges towards me and barks, then he's back below the bridge. Perhaps he was asking permission for a drink. He's back. More barking, dancing thrown in too, then back under the bridge. Just how he was with Paul in the forest. I can see him sniffing madly around the bank of the brook; clearly there have been dogs and people there, perhaps a massive scent dump. He's back, insistent, angrier, eyes boring command into me. Trust your dog.

Has he found a body, this early in the search? There's only us here. His bark rings in my ears as it bounces off the underside of the bridge. Maybe scent is coming downstream? Could be a body just out of area to see what I would do. Trust your dog.

Back on to the bridge for a better view upstream, my tension heading for the red zone. Nothing. Scout has followed me, really angry, bouncing up and down, then under the bridge, head around the parapet, his voice rolling downstream. He definitely wants me down there but doesn't want a drink. Someone is here, he's telling me, his face rising to the sky. Nothing hanging. As the bridge's shadows clear, right there, in between the bridge and its pier, is a man, grinning wildly, thumbs up. I'm so dumbstruck I forget to reward Scout. Trust your dog.

The body had been there an hour he tells me, rubbing life back into his legs, stomping his feet to get some warmth in. Scout had caught his scent cascading down, returned to me and would not give in. He'd found and stuck with it, trusting his nose, and me. It's a phenomenal find. I radio it in to Steve.

'See. Trust your dog.'

Buzzing with confidence we move on. I heap praise on Scout, who holds his head high with a big smile and chest out – king of the mountain.

We make our way through the boulder field, Scout pathfinding an easier route underfoot. The most efficient would be top to bottom, but that is a massive burn of energy for both of us; a thirty-degree slope and over 900 feet of ascent through heather and bracken is no gentle ramble. We need to keep a reserve for more searches. As we reach our northern boundary, we move higher and turn south, the wind now at our back. I maintain a straight line using boulders as aiming points, painting strips of cleared land across the hillside. Scout moves along and through my line, his favourite way of working, drawing a sine wave across the slope, any scent inside drawing into his nose. We've been working for forty minutes from the step on to the bridge when he turns sharply into a curve, picking his way to a narrow gully hidden by bracken. He works it through in his mind, moving this way and that in the scent cone, until I no longer see him. A minute, maybe two, the chimes falling silent, then I hear them again and see a channel being driven towards me. For a moment in the closeness of the stalks he loses me, jumps on to a rock, scans the hillside, his head giving a double take as he finds me, the surprise catching him. He locks my position, drops down and continues the tunnelling arriving at my feet, big bark, and back down the tunnel. When I arrive, there is the body smiling amongst a jumble of rocks.

Like this we work the land, breaking out above the bracken line to the crag of Indian's Head. Now in open land we move quickly and find a third body in a tiny cave. Scout is reluctant to go in. As I near, I see the reason –

the body is with his Border collie, both well known to us. The dog none too happy at Scout's presence, Scout exercises caution as the better part of valour.

I'm very satisfied with the whole exercise. Scout has proven his ability and I've quelled my worries about fitness. We take a few moments to sit on a rock and process the day. Two good search exercises, good finds, no issues. I'm happy.

Back at the Office, the debrief goes over the good and the bad. It's mostly good. That's the pre-assessment passed they tell me. I never knew. Come January we will be going for operational assessment in the Lake District. We are within touching distance of being a working search dog team.

Alan Rouse became the first British climber to summit K2, a tremendous achievement on that most difficult of mountains. Sadly, on the descent the team were trapped by a storm, only two of the seven surviving; Rouse was one who perished. He began climbing in the north-west of Britain, moving to Wales and eventually Sheffield for the gritstone and community of men and women married to rock. In preparation for K2, he devised a punishing training regime that included repeated ascents of Win Hill via Parkin Clough, a narrow, steep rocky ravine, carrying a pack full of rocks, returning from the summit with an empty pack to refill and repeat, over and over again.

Years later, on April Fool's Day, a local mountain rescue team instigated Rouse's route as a fitness test for team members, carrying full winter kit and completed in under thirty minutes, a distance of almost one kilometre with an ascent of 330 metres, almost a thirty-degree unrelenting climb. The record stands at nineteen minutes. It was said local gyms and slimming clubs around that time saw a significant uptick in membership while pub landlords gazed out at empty seats.

Cut Gate is an ancient drovers' route over the high moors connecting Yorkshire and Derbyshire; livestock, coal, iron and salt all moved along its six-kilometre length that rises 300 metres to the summit cairn. It is a wide track, easily visible on the ground with deep ruts and bogs in places. Compensating for its lack of steepness is the drudgery of a monotonous slog. In winter, the exposure across the barren windswept moor can easily snatch a life. In spring after rain and a winter of snow and ice, peat bogs can devour with impunity walkers' expensive boots, and cyclists' even more expensive mountain bikes. At night, the isolation is magical, surrounded as it is by cities of the industrial North; the summit cairn marks a black hole in the halo of light on the horizon. It is my own team's fitness test, ninety minutes in winter from the road to the cairn with full winter kit.

I have a few months to get us in peak condition. Scout is gaining strength from the tougher ground we now train on; his body ripples with muscle as the terrain hones power into him. Watching him flow through the landscape is to witness a shadow passing.

I begin a mix of strength, endurance and agility using the running track in the park along with the hills and boulder fields in the forest. My main concern is cardio; I need to increase my lung capacity and function as it often feels as though something is stopping my lungs from fully inflating. I reason this may be restricting the oxygen to my muscles, especially my legs. I've noticed when walking uphill others seem to cope better, hold conversations easily. I remain quiet, promising myself to eat more healthily. Parkin Clough and Cut Gate beckon. It's time to get the Ron Hill Tracksters out.

I hate running.

I run at night in the park, conscious of anyone seeing me. It's never elegant or inspirational, this old man, the young kids from the running club streaming past, some catching my shoulder in exasperation as they negotiate the slow-moving load. Scout keeps me company, albeit in front, beaming as young hands stroke him.

The weather is unusually benign following the long hot summer, making Cut Gate an easy if boring passage on my first attempt. I make it in sixty-four minutes and feel comfortable. Other team members take the test too; we pass one another, paying close attention to the pack size the other is carrying. I'm the fifth quickest in a team of fifty, not bad for an old man.

The park running and Cut Gate give me a baseline to measure progress. I choose a midweek afternoon to make my first attempt on Win Hill, reasoning there will be fewer people in the confines of Parkin Clough. If I need to bail early – which seems likely – I can, without anyone knowing. The clock begins with my hand on the bridge spanning the River Derwent, a short easy section of road, then wooden steps pulling at calves and glutes, the treads deep enough to burn thighs and trigger the first thoughts of giving up. I keep a steady pace, controlling my breathing as I burrow deeper into the hillside. Despite the season the clough feels oppressive, the humidity high in the sparse light which leaks through the canopy. The narrow path is a rocky, uneven surface creeping through tree roots and friable earth. A stream gurgles away on my left giving Scout plenty of cold water, and here and there a discarded plastic bottle. He drops the early one in my path but soon gets the message this is not play time and shifts his focus to scrambling up the stream. He is well ahead of me, choosing a line that is easy and comfortable, his body moving sweetly. I follow, ungainly, head down. When I look up, Scout is standing high above watching my progress with steady, knowing eyes; as the gap closes, he satisfies some thought and moves on. We pass through a wooden gate then the summit is one last push, a scramble up rock then across the flat hilltop to the trig pillar. Touch the concrete and hit the stopwatch, crumple in a heap on the cold triangulation pillar, feel my heart pounding, my lungs struggling for air. I'm beat. Scout sits looking, his tail hesitant. My time is twenty-nine minutes and forty-eight seconds.

Cut Gate I work once a month, Scout trotting happily in front. We beat the cut-off each time. I make it up Win Hill once a week with Scout watching. By the time Christmas comes I'm hitting the summit trig in twenty-three minutes.

There is frivolity about the place, the gathering for a weekend of training and laughter in the mountains of the Lake District. Anticipation is high for the Christmas meal, the hostel ablaze in the festivities. Happiness spreads to everyone after the recent assessment in Wales, all handlers passing on to the call-out list. I congratulate them, happy they made it. They can finally relax, moving easier, no longer carrying the weight of expectation and the long chain of doubt. After New Year, Scout and I will be casting off the same hard-forged shackles.

The weekend is the final phase for us, a time to attend to the last few percentages of improvement, enjoy our time on the hill while eyes watch closely, and not to get injured. I'm to bed early, Scout tucked up in the van, pyjamas on, warm blankets wrapping him in a cocoon of dreams. He's no inkling how momentous the coming weeks will be for us. Almost two and a half years to get here, from a cute puppy to a strong, gentle, intelligent working dog at ease anywhere. It's been a ride of elation and despair. But we are here.

Of the three of us who began training, two of us will be taking the assessment. The Third Man has seen a change in fortunes, spending the days isolated with his dog trying to fix the latest problem. The tougher it has become for him the more he has retreated into himself. I try to bring him into the fold, asking how the day has gone; he doesn't answer. I tell him to take care, things will get better.

The only thing that can stop us now is a sheep chase, the great fear of handlers. In our time several dogs have succumbed to temptation, all have quietly moved on to spend life by the fire as the family pet. Just a few months from assessment a dog launched itself out of a van, bounded across the moor in hot pursuit of a flock of sheep that was pouring over the horizon, the handler in frantic pursuit screaming expletives to no avail as dog and sheep vanished. The sheep were safe. All knew the outcome for dog and handler, everyone secretly pleased it was not their dog. Finally, dog, now leashed, and handler took the lonely walk back to the van, neither making eye contact with each other or anyone else. No one moved to offer a comforting word. The silently condemned drove off in the same direction the sheep had sought refuge, the sheep now long gone, the van bumping its slow misery and tears down the rough track. They would not return.

While I trust Scout implicitly, I watch carefully – trust but verify. It is not the flock that is the worry, it's the lone sheep dozing unseen, unexpectedly surprised by Scout, the pair scared half witless by the encounter, the sheep legging it in panic, and Scout thinking, *righto, playtime*.

I lie in my bunk and push the image away from sleep.

Gray Crag is steep and keeps getting steeper. It tests a handler's ability in vertiginous terrain and inclement weather. The dog will move comfortably with their four-by-paw drivetrain. There is no bracken; yellowing grass has a clear sweep from Pasture Beck to the crag line, a wall of silver-grey rock, beyond that, the deepening black of a winter sky. There's the wet shading of isolated rowan, the odd Herdwick amongst boulders of pink granite. Patches of sharp, unstable grey scree will extract huge amounts of energy as stones slip from under hard boots – at first a pleasing tapping of stonechat rolling softly down the scree field, then unsettlingly the sound of a drum roll, then snare drum rattle as the mass slips above and below in an unstoppable multitude of tiny avalanches that engulf anything in their path. With relief trickling to a quiet stop. There is a tendency to drift down as one traverses, people taking the easier, softer way, ambling off course, swathes of an area missed. Fix a point ahead and keep your eye on it.

A finger traces the outline of a box from one prominent feature to the next. Pasture Beck the base, sky top, right hand a gully, left hand a shaky finger and a description that trails across England. I reckon I can work it out when I get there and say nothing. The wind is screaming down the walls, dark opaque clouds settling as they prepare to dump snow. It's cold, the wind whipping any degree of warmth out of the day, the air stubbornly a centimetre or two below zero. I lay out my plan. Split the area in two, zigzag up the left, across the top, zigzag down the right to the bottom and out of the search exercise. Simple and efficient. The steepness will burn large amounts of fuel in both of us so how I manage our energy will be an important indicator if we cover this area in our January assessment. There are lots of technical locations – crags, hollows, water, places where scent can settle or swirl around – and ground to pause for thought and think how to traverse without becoming the casualty. A few hours of enjoyment.

There is major rivalry between the handlers of Border collies, and those with other dogs, especially Spanners (spaniels). Which is best. The answer obvious to each side. You have to be fit for a Spanner, the things running around like demented clockwork mice, consuming land at a ridiculous rate. Border collies are more methodical, cleverer, work much harder and for much longer. Because of this, it is the more intelligent, technically gifted handler who has a Border collie. So they say.

Scout settles himself while I adjust my pack. I take a photograph of the area for my record along with the map I have drawn, my route detailing any markers. I have my radio; the phone is only for reference, there's no signal here in this vast bowl, and it isn't permitted to use GPS to track my progress. I need to show awareness of the ground covered; the phone stays in my salopettes pocket.

By zigzagging through the area, I can push Scout out to the flanks covering more ground without having to myself. The secret is to give Scout enough rest; a handler has advised me to rest for a short time every twenty minutes. I set an alarm on my phone. At twenty minutes we reach a scrape halfway up; Scout lies down in the bowl away from the wind. We're both super relaxed and working well. I reset the phone, share water, and nibble: flapjack for me, pemmican – a dense bar with high fat content, the same fuel that they take on Antarctic adventures – for Scout. The next stop is the summit.

Four walkers pass above, their bodies braced against the wind howling over the crag. We'd passed a scrape a few metres below and decamp there, putting my pack down on the lip of the scrape for protection; Scout watches every move. I bunker down; the higher we've climbed the more the weather has deteriorated, the snow tipping beyond its threat; flurries of large flakes sweep over the crag, swirling into the valley like a scattering of grain. People below look small, the stream a pencil line. As I open my pack a blast of wind rocks it forwards; my hat and sandwich box cartwheel into the 900-foot void, the plastic box spinning, hitting rock, then jettisoning out into the emptiness getting smaller and smaller as it laughs at me. My hat, caught by the wind, floats and twirls through eddies of snowflakes, the beauty of its movement mesmerising until it drifts over a rocky knoll and is lost. I debate whether to go down – 900 feet down and 900 feet back up. The radio crackles into life, a voice saying this is an area of outstanding natural beauty, all litter should be taken home. I can see half a dozen red jackets pointing binoculars at me. They'll be laughing for sure. I give them two fingers and turn away to check the time on my phone. It isn't there.

I cannot believe how inept I've been. Dragging myself into self-recrimination I fail to get the body on the left-hand boundary, not going far enough, even when Scout shows definite interest. I find later the body is out of area, which is a small crumb of comfort. We head across the top and down to traverse the scree field. The stones are very sharp, and I fear for Scout's pads. He's having an issue with stones moving underneath his paws; I can see him trying to work out a strategy to deal with the strange surface. Gradually, he gravitates towards the edges where the soft grass is stable and easier on the paws. I get his plan, directing him around the swatch of stone; calculating the strong wind will drive any scent towards him, while I can clearly see the grey mass, and any human from higher up. Clearing the scree we move through easier ground of sheep-shorn grass.

Scout goes into a deep cleft, straight up a little brook tumbling over a series of rocky ledges, slippery with moss and greasy rock; he moves deeper into the mountain the higher he reaches. Old rowan cling to thin soil and rise out of cracked stone. Scout vanishes into the darkness. I hear the tinkling of his bell and the babble of the water. Then a long silence. I stand and peer into the blackness. His shape emerges; he indicates and tells me to follow. It's a good find with lots happening to muddy the scent. The position of the body explains the long silence: to get down I have to be really careful on the slippery rock; to get back out I'm in danger of needing rescue. Scout watches me closely. He's already skipped up the smaller rocks and pulled himself out. Doesn't take his eyes off me or what I'm grabbing. My hand finds a small hold that will take my weight; he doesn't seem sure, huffing and puffing as he examines it. I give it a big tug and it flies off, my body swinging around with the momentum of my pack; Scout barks and begins to descend. 'I'm okay,' I tell him, 'stay there.' My boot finds a hold and I take an extra big step up, caution to the wind. Scout grabs my pack with his teeth, his soft lips and saliva hot on my freezing head. Eventually I make it, lie on the ground fingers red and cold, Scout's front paws on my chest, his face rolling down to me, the long pink tongue licking my face.

We move on and find the third body behind a wall by the stream, then we are out and finished, rewarded by a warming sun from a washed blue sky. I feel good despite the fiasco at the beginning – almost three hours in the area, a tough session, a little dignity lost, our fitness tested and not found wanting. I prepare myself for the inevitable humiliation. They do not disappoint, asking what I've got for lunch, and should I be wearing a hat to keep the brain working. I don't mention the phone.

I make a mistake that evening. Needing to talk to Alison, I ask a handler if I can use his phone. This is the mistake.

'Why?'

I'm an idiot. Committed, I tell him about losing my phone on the exercise. His grin is broad, his face beaming. He ensures everyone in the room knows, skipping down corridors to spread the delightful news. I make the call.

Fifteen minutes later he's back brandishing a text from Alison who has located my phone with a finder app. The irony is not lost on me. It's on the hillside where I took the photo of Scout. The handler, young, keen as mustard, yet to have a find, causing him some angst – he and his dog will save someone's life in time to come – offers to go and find it with his Border collie. One of the bodies says he'll come too. There's a hooley blowing outside, the storm well dug in for the night; sleet lashes down in great sheets hammering the glass and rattling window frames, spreading a frozen white mush on the ground. He's excited. I say yes. We head out through the silent narrow lanes then a rough track until a raging stream blocks the way. Fording the water crashing through swollen falls, feet skidding on slippery rock, we make it to the foot of Gray Crag. The snow is hard, translucent ice from livestock hooves twisting ankles and ripping feet from underneath our bodies battling against the rage of the wind. Even with goggles it's hard to see; the snow zips past like shooting stars in the light from our head torches, the wind pulls and pushes. The handler directs his dog around where Alison said, but the fierce wind denies it any scent from the phone. After an hour I say we should get back inside; I can feel the disappointment on his face.

Next morning, we are in the same valley to train, which is odd because we've never trained in the same place twice. There are a lot more dogs and handlers; some arrived last night, but there still seems too many. I can feel a furtiveness around, little groups holding whispered discussions.

The Second Man I started obedience class with is already out on the hill, moving quickly, his dog zipping about, tail wagging furiously, working the same ground we worked yesterday. My radio fires into life and his voice asks if my phone was a feminine gold iPhone. It is, I meekly admit. Silence. Then he tells me his dog has found it. His dog, a Spanner, has found my phone. It's a crushing defeat, applauded by a huge roar around the valley as everyone joins in my humiliation. I will never live this moment down. Never be allowed to forget it. The great divide between Border collie and spaniel handlers just got wider to the detriment of collies. I'm crestfallen. The phone still works.

Scout and I are next. The bodies are probably in different places, but conditions are the same, though now there is snow and ice on the slope. We will follow yesterday's plan. Near a small knoll Scout picks up scent on the wind and takes off along a small crag. Minutes later he is back demanding my attendance. As I reach the spot, he is standing there, but no body. 'Show me.' I'm thinking the body might be in a scrape I cannot see yet; he gives me a look of pained despair, dips his head into some long grass and pulls out my hat and begins juggling. It's a great find. Up on that cold, windswept crag with my hat jumping up and down in the blue sky, I know he's telling me I let him down yesterday. He's chastising me, telling me to get my act together because we can do this. That's what he tells me.

I never find the sandwich box, never know what filling I had ordered. That evening we gather for Christmas dinner, a throng of people in tasteless jumpers, paper hats askew, streamers floating across tables, the end of another year. The last few days have helped me be part of this community more than I realised I needed to be. I was touched by the offer of help in that raging storm, touched by all the laughter at my expense.

Tomorrow, we make the journey home, the same route we took two and half years ago when Scout was cradled in the palm of my hand, swaddled in an old shirt with my scent, his beautiful face, those pink paws, that puppy smell, the deep cosmos of his eyes drawing me in.

In four weeks, we will be here again for our operational assessment; everything is in place. Looking around at all the smiling faces listening to the banter and the jokes, there is a happy goodwill. Of the three of us from the Peak District, two of us have made it to the final stage. There is not a single person in the room who has not had some input in our progress. The lessons I have learned, tempered with knowledge and experience, have been freely given from this disparate group of handlers and dogsbodies. Without Steve, we would not be here. I know our goal is attainable, and I'm certain this is the contribution we are meant to be making. The fantasy of being a dog handler on the hill has been replaced by the reality of being a dog team. And I am no longer alone, I am with Scout.

. . .

We are in a fallow time. The days spent in endless waiting, the landscape hibernating. In the forest there is more sky between the beech and pine, boots gather loamy earth to bring home, everything stretches into a grey dreariness. We've stopped training to prevent any injury, my biggest fear now we are so close. We walk the forest and moors on well-made paths, stay clear of livestock, ease down after the long period of training until we gently tick over, sit, talk, watch the leaves chase each other around.

We hammer up Parkin Clough once a week, three times each visit; my quickest time from bridge to trig is twenty-three minutes and forty seconds. Scout always ahead, his haunches bulging with power, making easy work of the steep rocky path. He stops now and again, interrupted by walkers who fuss him energetically while placing a worrying eye on me with my plodding approach, body heaving, face red, gasping for air.

The rest of the time we relax, work on basic obedience, have fun with the ball in the park. I drive up to the Lakes with the Second Man to look at possible assessment areas: typical mountain landscape, glacial valleys, streams, walled green fields low down reaching up to the brown bracken line; boulders sit randomly where they rested hundreds of millions of years ago, gullies slice upward to a grey line of crag and on to the sky. Green, brown, grey. On the day, hopefully lots of blue. That's the colour scheme we want. We don't want white. Snow will sap energy. Harder for bodies too, who have to walk circuitous routes to their bivvy location without leaving a line of footprints, leaving handlers kicking their heels in a lay-by, waiting. We don't want fog, low cloud, mist, call it what you will. Poor visibility means the team has a watcher dogging each step right behind them, slowing them down, adding new levels of stress to an already stressful day. We hope for colourful days with a blue top.

The assessment is by formal invitation. Waiting for the email becomes the focus of my day. I check my inbox daily, hourly, every few minutes, sending numerous emails to myself convinced Google has chosen to disconnect my account, just mine, at just this moment. Refreshing the page, I hold my breath as the download hangs, watch the little lights on the router blink on and off, exhale disappointedly when I see spam offering me a cheap holiday in the summer sun. Finally, the invite arrives. I sit looking at the bold subject line as Dad's clock ticks seconds of life away, then call Alison. Both of us sit watching the little hand hover over the line, then click, a whole page fills the screen with words we read aloud again and again. I have to RSVP. It takes seconds to confirm Scout and I will be in attendance. Now sit back, hold hands with Alison and stare at the screen. Scout, Monty and Olly join us, not wanting to miss anything, the house suddenly empty of their humans. Scout lies behind, making happy grumbling noises, gazing at his favourite toy in his paws high above him.

I book accommodation. I don't want the free bed waiting for me, don't want to be near the constant glare. The other handler does the same. Then a twilight world of nothingness, the days holding on to the hours until the moon signals the turning to summer. I study scenarios, spending hours looking at the photos of the terrain, trying to read the narrative of the land, find a way of communicating with it. I pack, repack, and pack again, charge batteries several times, buy stuff off the internet I have never needed and never will, in the knowledge that these items are essential to stave off failure. Alison tiptoes across fields of eggshells on every floor. Sinews and fibres draw tighter and tighter, my skin taut, the air at home creaking with the strain of creeping tension.

Not knowing how we will be measured in the assessment becomes my new obsession. I try to discuss it with Steve, other handlers, but all I get are mixed messages that trail off into ifs and buts. Not knowing is hard. Backing myself into a corner I open up to Alison, show her how vulnerable I am. She listens, then counsels. Scout and I can only do our best, and we will. Keep it simple.

WINTER AND SPRING 2019

As the new year slips in we take long walks through the forest, keeping to the trails, away from other dogs, sheep and cows. With a few days to go, the other handler pulls out as his dog is injured. Three years of work halted in one moment. I feel for them. We're on our own, the only survivors of obedience class.

Home is spiky with static, childish excitement and rigid conformity. Hard to believe we are doing this. Three years of work ends with five mountain searches over one weekend. Madness. We take a final walk to relax, letting Scout root around quiet forest trails. He's so carefree, completely in the moment, finding sticks, hunting down scent dumps, romping through his favourite waterfall trying to catch silver bubbles. Snow hangs over the edge of the stream, the sun catching the marriage of snow, ice and water, uncovering glimpses of sparkling diamonds. I call him out, slip his lead on and head for home.

That evening the house tries to relax, I read and read the same words, Alison watches a film, staying quiet, Monty and Olly doze, Scout lies on his bed cleaning his paws. It's a long night, hours staring into space, going over search areas, strategies, things I might have forgotten. I check the time, check again, my world still held by the night. We'll travel at 11 a.m. – a gentle drive to soothe nerves, try to enjoy the journey. I listen to Alison's breathing, feeling the regular rhythm through the darkness. Gradually, the edges of the windows grow light. Our day is here.

The tappity click of paws from downstairs announces the dogs wanting breakfast. I slip out of bed without disturbing Alison. All three dogs greet me, Monty pushing to the front for the biggest slice of attention, Olly at the

121

back being good, Scout edging towards the stairs to be first into the kitchen. I go to the bathroom first, they all follow, stretch themselves out on the heated floor. When I leave, they rattle down the stairs, yelping to each other in excitement. I follow, telling them to be quiet. I notice red spots. Wet, lurid and shiny on the oak floor. I can't think if they were there before. There's more on the stairs, and the ground floor. The dogs are dancing around wanting their food, and blood is smearing everywhere. I bellow for Alison, grab Monty who has a habit of knocking his tail till it bleeds. Nothing. Then Scout whose long tongue lolling lengthily out of his mouth often gets bitten. Nothing. Olly looks good. But the blood is still coming. I shout the dogs to be still. Monty and Olly head under the table. Scout sits in his bed and licks his paw, a pink stain of skin on his white socks. It's blood. It runs down my hand as I hold his paw. A pad is cut, deep, something that will need the vet before we set off for assessment. Behind me Alison holds her head.

The vet gives us the news. The cut is deep, will need stitches and at least a month of rest. I ask if he can still do the assessment. No.

There are only two assessments a year, November and tomorrow. It will be ten months until our next opportunity. We will not be getting operational status in a few days' time. It's over.

Over the coming days my emotions find a place to settle. At home Scout limps around; a sky-blue bandage with cartoon dogs protects his paw. He climbs on to the settee to spend the evenings cuddling, a rare treat from him. He can't go for walks. I go into the forest alone, feeling the emptiness where my best friend should be. The snow has melted; his waterfall still runs black. Something glitters. I bend to pick it up, get a sharp pain, see blood mix with the cold black water. Between my thumb and finger is a bright piece of glass. I make an oath to Scout.

Scout languishes mournfully in bed. He lies in idle stupor, chin resting on his favourite toy, his eyes absorbing the household. To be restricted to the house must seem a punishment. I spend evenings talking softly to him, but he still wallows in self-pity.

In the third week the stitches come out – the wound is beautifully healed. I take no chances, lead walking the next few days, getting move-ment and flex back into his paw. He's happy to be out, making long stops to check out his social media sites, updating with his downloads – 'I'm back.' I scan ahead for anything sharp, check his paws after every walk. By mid-February we are back on the hill.

Scout is in fine spirit and form; the more we work the better he gets.

His strike distance is now so great he spends long periods out of my sight. His indication is more insistent, brutal. He hunts down the source of scent, analysing, discarding, moving ahead in and out of the ever-narrowing cone. Running through his binary sampling, the neurons clicking through all the permutations – here, not here, stronger. Then thundering back to me, obstacles given passing contempt, a face completely absorbed, his message delivered with rock-shattering force: 'I've found. Move it.' He keeps this going to and fro between me and the source until I am with him, his head high, haughty, tail bashing furiously through vegetation, beams shooting out from every fibre, eyes boring into my pocket.

I'm different too. The ground seems easier, our communication seamless. I can direct with a whistle, an outstretched hand, a few paces in a particular direction. We spend joyous hours on the hill.

In March, we get chance of an operational assessment in a few weeks' time piggy-backed on to the Welsh dogs' test weekend. I accept immediately.

The operational assessment is on the last weekend in April – a small gathering of dogs, including the Second Man who missed out through injury last time. Of the Third Man and dog, there has been no sign.

The forecast says it will be clear and mild, with a nice easy breeze.

The assessment briefing answers all the questions I had: criteria, time, indication, control, coverage; there is nothing of concern. We need four passes out of five areas over the three days.

The first day we are in the mountains at Cwm Gwdi, an old army camp, the buildings long gone. I'm more nervous than I expected as I outline my plan to the assessors. Take the left-hand boundary that will be collecting all the scent, work up to the top of the hill, then zigzag back down. We've two hours to complete. It's 10:30 a.m. and the clock starts.

I'm wearing compression socks to help the blood flow in my legs; they've been getting heavier lately – that lack of oxygen – and right now I'm trying to get as much air into my tense chest as I can. We enter the centre of the bottom boundary; the left-hand boundary looks steeper from here, time-consuming and exhausting if I don't settle myself down. The right-hand boundary curves gently up through a gully opening out below the skyline where it gets steep. I slip Scout's coat on, 'Find him out.' He does his song and dance then disappears into a patch of gorse. There are sheep around and a little shiver runs through me. He's back, and no sheep heading for the horizon as he barrels to me, indicates, spins around. I pick my way along, arms in the air trying to avoid thorns; when I reach him, he's sitting proudly by the first body. I gush over him with pleasure and no small amount of surprise. Trust your dog. It's 10.40 a.m.

My breathing wrong-foots me. I think it best I take the easier right-hand boundary to the top. We head into the wind clearing out a wide strip of land to the gully. I've made a mistake not calling in the change of plan, but I'm so happy at the early find I am oblivious to the error.

I give Scout a chunk of pemmican then send him in an arc around the bottom of the gully. As he circles through the wind, first heading downwind then turning into the stream again, he shoots down a grassy bank, springs back out and tells me he has had another find. Sure enough there is the second body with Scout beaming beside him. Trust your dog. It is 11.15 a.m.

A steady ascent gets us to the top of the hill. We work back to the collecting boundary, the ground passing under our feet quickly, letting the exertion of the climb ease out of my legs and lungs.

Near the left-hand boundary Scout turns back into the wind, scrambling down to find the third body under a ledge, then scrambling back up, all excited, to tell me. Trust your dog. It is 11.55 a.m.

I radio in the find; tell them I will continue working my way down to clear the rest of the land. As we drop down, I get the call to come out. We have finished. I'm pleased: three bodies found, area cleared, well within time. I slip Scout's coat off to let him know we have finished and tease him with some treats, smother him in kisses, ready to hear how well we did.

'Why didn't you work from the collecting boundary?' the two assessors ask. I stand my ground, tell them about the easier route on the right, about conserving energy. They listen, say nothing. I do not mention the breathing.

The second area is smaller, more intricate. There are crags, false summits, gullies. And sheep. It is 2 p.m.

The wind tumbles straight down to us as we work into the landscape, taking the left-hand side first, aiming for the top, then back down the right-hand side. Scout gets an immediate note of scent and clambers his way into a boulder-strewn gully. I let him work at his pace. There's gorse and bits of heather, gnarled hawthorn, remnants of brick buildings, all clinging to a meagre soil. The sound of his bell sparkles in the sunlight, then he appears, rushing down to me. I can see his mind saying over and over: *I've found, tell him I've found.* I pick my way through the rock to a tunnel running into the hillside, with Scout and the first body. Great find. The body, hidden inside a drift mine, is in a stream of super-chilled air rising from the depths of the earth. Trust your dog. It is 2.30 p.m.

We've climbed a few hundred metres; I decide to keep my height and work to the top, taking in the higher reaches of the left-hand boundary, then across a ridge and down the right-hand boundary. Scout quarters the land clearing vast areas of space until he indicates another find in open ground. I cannot see anything, other than Scout next to some flattened brown bracken. He holds his ground. 'Show me then.' He looks at me in despair, points his nose to the ground. Just a mass of rotting bracken on yellow grass. Another look at me, then the bracken. I give in, kick some of the bracken away and a boot comes into view. 'Good boy,' I shout. The body springs from its winter hibernation. Trust your dog. It is 3.15 p.m.

I radio in, tell them what we have left to do; they tell me to come out. The assessors ask if I have covered it all. I say about the bit on the right I had to clear after the final find. 'What about the bottom left-hand corner?' they ask. The piece of ground below where I decided to keep my height after the first find. What is wrong with me? 'It's okay,' they say, 'it's within the allowable tolerance.' One assessor, a gentle Scottish man – studied, well respected, preferring his own company – says 'you have been the only team to find the body under the bracken. You've passed, but don't make a habit of missing bits. Draw the area out and tick searched sections off as you go.'

We get two area passes, three more to go. The next day will include the area that forced the handler to abandon the assessment all those years back when I was a body. For us, there's been a good stretch of dry weather, streams will be lower and the rock dry. All we have to do is take our time and work the plan. I talk through the day with Steve. He's out of the national mix now, just working his dog for his own team, training any handlers that ask for help. I've stayed with him because I respect him, he's never led me astray, always been straight and honest; that's as good as it gets for me. He already knows most of my day, the whispers going north. 'You've passed two areas,' he tells me. 'Tomorrow take your time and stay calm. Watch your coverage and if you get dragged off route make sure you go back, mark the spot, with your pack if you must. You know all this. We both know you and Scout can do it, so enjoy it. Remember: trust your dog.'

Later I speak to Alison; I don't mention mistakes, just that we have passed both areas and Scout is doing well. For dinner I add sardines to Scout's bowl. During the night, the weather shifts.

Our third area, Y Gyrn, has swirling wind and driven snow. It is 10.30 a.m.

Scout is in his element. The humpback hill is tough ground with pockets of Welsh sheep sheltering from the weather. We work methodically as Steve taught, meticulous on coverage, sketching the area in my notebook, shading those cleared as we go, the hit of adrenaline pushing out the nerves.

The first body is just below the top of the hill, the westerly lifting the scent over the ridge into Scout's nose. He'd scrambled down, sprung back up, and there he was. A simple clean find. Trust your dog. It is 11.10 a.m.

We stick to the plan taking a break by a large boulder. The wind's swung round to an easterly now. Scout clears snow from his paws; I check my map. After two minutes we continue. I'm unaware that thirty metres west of the boulder, downwind, is a body. As we pass back below the body the wind is westerly. We are almost finished, and we've only found one body, a thought I try to push away. The wind switches again, the easterly pulling Scout up to a gnarled blackthorn. He returns, indicates, he's found. Trust your dog. It is 12.15 p.m.

I radio in – they say I'm finished and to bring the body out with me. She was born inside a Welsh mountain – tough and fast. I'm out of breath trying to keep my end of the conversation going. She asks if we found her husband.

'At the top,' I say.

'No, in the middle,' she glances. I'm silent. The assessors explain about the change in wind direction, just bad luck, not a fail to find. We pass with high marks.

I'm pleased how we both worked, a real team effort, and we're enjoying the day. Scout has a broad smile, his nose pecking at the smell of bacon. Why not.

The fourth area is the vertical crag with the traversing ledges, Craig y Fro; it is known as RAC Technical, the name raising fear in many handlers. 'Technical' because of the difficulty of the terrain and what it does to scent: all those faces, gullies and waterfalls forming countless eddies, dumps of scent dropped like a stone. And its exposure, inducing fear in handler and dog. 'RAC' because a breakdown patrol used to park opposite in a large lay-by, waiting for trouble on the long pull out of the valley on the A470 from Brecon. In its position now is the butty wagon.

From the lay-by the public enjoy a good view of the area, dog and handler, likening the crags to the North Face of the Eiger. There is danger; no one in their right mind would cross this crag, and never in bad weather. It splits into a series of shelves, black rock and grass strewn with debris from the face. One side is the crag, the other, unrelenting exposure. Three black gullies drive vertically, dividing the face, water thundering over the ledges with winter melt. The base of the crag runs out on to scree, then grass, then road. The odd blackthorn adds interest, but everyone looks at the crag and the crashing waters.

The afternoon sun adds snowmelt to the waters falling down the permanent shadow of the cold crag's north-east face; a screeching wind spirals up the rock, spray lifting into the airy space for a bone-chilling soak. The plan is to search from bottom to top; any way will mean getting cold and wet. The menacing effect of gravity, the crashing cymbals and the slippery rock create a sublime theatre of awe and horror. It is the first time I have searched in my helmet. Scout gives me a double take, then sniffs the wind. It is 2 p.m.

He heads for the first gully. I encourage him up, my voice as light as I can risk over the drum kit blaring out from the chasm. Behind a blackthorn, I can just hear his bell; now he's back with a big smile on his face; it's a favourite body. He's excited and happy picking his way back across the water. Trust your dog. It is 2.20 p.m.

The snow has stopped falling, there's a blue sky and a sharp wind. It's glorious. We climb higher and traverse a ledge on the crag face, slippery with snow. I slow down; Scout engages full four-by-paw, scrambles down fifty metres, his body articulating through boulders, comes back, tells me he's found the second body. It's the husband of the first. Trust your dog. It is 2.50 p.m.

We've reached the technical bit, the gullies deep and vertical; scent rafts will be layering on a multitude of surfaces, carried by water and wind. Crossing the gullies means a series of ascents and descents along ledges and ground strewn with shifting stone. Scout skips across and waits, checking I'm safe. I take my time, not even getting my boots wet. When I reach him, I take a moment to steady myself; he keeps his gaze on my eyes. *'You okay?'* I actually tell him, 'Yes, I'm okay,' and give him a stroke. He gives me the once over then moves on. The wind changes direction pouring over the top of the crag; flakes of snow swirl between huge dumps of water as the chain gets pulled above us. We hold position until the anger subsides.

The wind swings round to an easterly, coming up to meet us. Two thirds of the way across Scout sticks his nose into the void and begins picking his way down the gully, stepping carefully, an avalanche of small stones running out ahead of him. He stops occasionally to survey the route, looks back to check on me. Boulders move him off course, but he works hard to regain the scent cone, inching forwards as the strength of the cone increases, then continues his descent. Almost at the bottom he merges into the trees where our first body is hiding. Scout pops out, scans the crag face; when he has my position, he begins his ascent to me. I drop my pack off at the spot and begin my descent, giving him the respect he has earned. I can see he is tiring of all the climbing, but he still gives a full indication, spins around and guides me into the body. Trust your dog. It is 3.15 p.m.

She's laughing her head off at me having to come all the way back down. We have a long rest, we have time. I radio in the find and give them my plan. We slog back up to my pack and continue across the face to exit overlooking the last gully. This one is wide, more grass and less rock. Scout is pulled all the way down to where we entered the area, then disappears from view. Minutes pass; I cannot decide to stay or go down, I'm sure he has found, but the thought of climbing down and back up again isn't enticing. I spot him on the other side of the gully staring at me. He's not sure. He makes his way up one hell of a pull and still has enough energy to do his routine. *'I've found some scent but there isn't a body. I need your help.'* I follow, encouraging him with happy words. At the edge of the gully his eyes drag mine down to the stream, eyebrows raised. *'See, nothing.'*

The wind is flowing uphill; that's what pulled him down. He has the scent, knows something is here but can't find the edges of the cone. I work him upstream and along the opposite bank where he scrambles out of sight, his bell telling me he's there. It's a long time before Scout climbs out, looks for me, then makes his way back to tell me he has found. I follow him back. There is a large overhang with a big drop I can't see the bottom of. I retrace my steps then work my way back up, asking Scout to speak so I can gauge how far I have to go. Behind a gnarly old tree anchored to a large rock, I see the body smiling. It's a magnificent result for Scout – he worked hard for a textbook find. Trust your dog. It is 3.40 p.m.

I radio in and tell the assessors what I have left, across the top and down for a nice easy exit, hoping they'll pull us out. No such luck, either there's another body, or they want their fun. We set off for the top; after five minutes slogging and cursing they tell me to come out. We've finished. Scout, his coat off, skips happily around the area, knowing he won't have to work again. At debrief the assessor says she's wasted her time if I am going to ignore everything she taught me. I'm at a loss to know what I have done wrong. The second assessor shows me the marking sheet, nine out of ten; it was a joy to watch they say. We celebrate with a bacon sandwich each.

We are awarded two more passes, just one more area to make sure. Only a sheep chase could deny us now, and I have no expectations that will happen. Scout gets more sardines in his dinner. I slip on compression socks and get to sleep.

A need for the bathroom has me up in the cold dark. At the top of the stairs, I slip; my feet and legs whipping out ahead of me, I miss all the steps bar the final one, landing heavily on my backside, the soft tissue creasing into the aluminium edge, my foot trapping beneath me as my weight and momentum slam me into a wall. The darkness envelops me.

Back in the light again, I lie quietly, trying to work out the injuries and think what to do. Minutes pass, the pain is coursing around my legs and body, my head vibrates and creaks, and I'm cold. My knee is tight but not broken. My glutes have a big dent the shape of the bottom step and possibly crushed muscle, tissue and probably nerves; it feels numb. I manage to crawl back to the bedroom, lying as still as possible on my back. My room-mate, the Second Man, sleeps soundly. If I cannot move tomorrow, we will have to pull out and we won't pass. I made an oath to Scout.

Morning comes. I'm stiff and in pain but moving. I dose myself up with painkillers and say nothing. The Second Man asks me if I heard a bump in the night; I tell him the tale, show him the bruising, spend minutes detailing the pain. You just need to man the fuck up, he says.

We are on the west side of Beacons Reservoir for the final area. The first body found after thirty minutes, the second and final within the hour. It's the body who was lying under the bracken on the first day. Today he was idling on the side of a gully. Trust your dog. It is 11.30 a.m.

I'm relieved it's all over. Everyone gathers to see us awarded the status of handler and search dog. We take our place on the call-out list.

It is 1 p.m. on 28 April 2019, exactly three years to the day and time since Scout joined our family.

We have made it.

The drive home is full of smiles, me telling Scout how proud I am of him, throwing him treats every few miles. When we walk in the door the house explodes in movement and noise, and treats; Monty and Olly join Scout dancing with Alison, I stand and take it all in. Until the phone goes.

It's a call-out, for dogs. Our first operational job. I'm bouncing around like an unstable atom, Alison is rushing to get food and drink ready, I'm fiddling with Scout's red operational search dog tag, and trying to get his new operational coat to fit. He looks so clean-cut, so professional. The Second Man and his dog, as new as us, are on their way, and closer too. To get a find within a few hours of passing the assessment would be a fairytale start to our careers. I thread through narrow streets to the Manchester Road. As we cross into the Peak District we're stood down; the missing person has turned up. I take a slow route back home, still feeling the adrenaline, still smiling. So, this is what it is like.

At team training, people congratulate Scout, slip him a biscuit or two from the barrel. We head out on our first team exercise as an operational dog team. It feels good. The team runs through a rope exercise. Scout relaxes on a rock watching the knitting, getting bored and dozing off. As the light fades, we step into our place within the team. It feels special, is special.

At Chew Valley, there's pats on the back, compliments to Scout for pulling me through; Steve quietly says well done. He never doubted.

Scout looks smart in his working jacket, the words *Mountain Rescue Search Dog*, the bell tinkling away, lights bouncing. Below his chin, set against his brilliant white fur rests the red dog tag denoting he is a qualified mountain rescue search dog. This one is special, made for him by his metal-smith mum. He looks perfect.

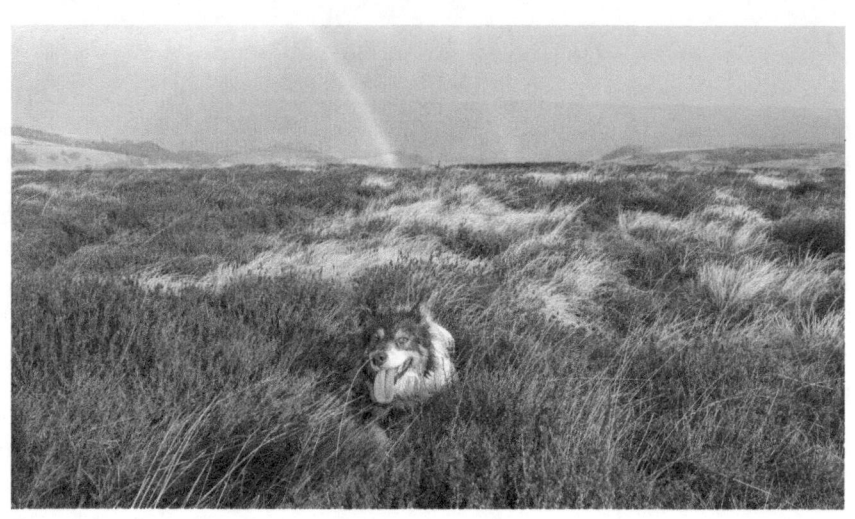

THE FIND

SUMMER AND AUTUMN 2019

The sun hangs veiled in thin cloud. The car park is full of vans. Young and middle-aged stare at phones, checking routes, times, statistics, tech engaging with the outdoors via apps and websites, performance measured against others, their own personal best against the world.

The newbie stands back from the group, nervous, the shiny bike protecting him. He's cajoled on to a track, his stomach churning. Older riders – men, always men – keep time at bay wearing tighter, brighter clothing, multiple pudgy rolls of beer and fry-ups showing the futility of it all. They tinker with brakes and gears, wrestle on carbon fibre armour while listening to the latest domestic from the thrice-married architect. I'm told, I wouldn't know, there are some world-class tracks running through the old woodland, fast and furious.

We're fortunate in the city to have so much green space. It's a mecca for outdoor activities, drawing people to study, work, live. The tracks have become a regular call-out for my team; we even have our own car park. It's mainly extraction work to waiting ambulances, the ground beyond anything the paramedics can deal with. If the team doctors and medics are lucky, they get there before the paramedics and have the chance to pull bones apart, reset, whack in some morphine, deal with a pneumothorax using a bit of bandage wrapper and some adhesive plasters. Injuries can be serious, the body rearranged as it hit the immovable object at high speed, the instant deceleration ripping through the frail human container. It can be life-threatening, even with a casualty sat upright talking calmly about what happened, friends looking on holding what's left of the bike, the injured quietly bleeding to death inside. We load and go over rough ground quickly, mummifying the casualty in vacuum-packed sleeping bags to prevent further trauma, two red lines either side of the stretcher, passing the casualty on in no worse state than when we all first met.

Scout attends all call-outs now. We think we know where the casualty is, but you cannot be sure until you are with them. Woodland paths can be deceptive, one tree looking like any other. If we aren't needed, he spends his time watching the comings and goings of the incident site, grabs attention from the bystanders keeping them out of the way. A call-out to a cardiac arrest high on the moor has Scout employed calming the casualty while awaiting the helicopter.

Scout gambols happily in his own world, exploring the life of the forest. It is serene, the sounds of nature surrounding us as we walk to see cow and calf in the pasture. Scout pecks away above the fence; they must be deeper in, the high bracken hiding them. When dogs and horses approach us, I call Scout. He closes in transferring his attention to a plastic water stillage, probably the scent of a cattleman. He pays the others a passing glance then drops into a stream, barely a trickle it's been so dry. I tell him to drink while I look for the birds I hear. I'm rubbish at this; I'm told to look for what should not be there but all I see are leaves and they all look the same.

Ahead Wharncliffe Chase runs to the horizon through moorland, crag and ancient deer park. It has a dragon who has a cave and damsels in distress on training nights. The cloud has burnt away, the insects are buzzing, it's getting warm. Scout now has to wait for the command entering water after the assessment debacle. I let him go and he chases bubbles jogging along the thin surface.

We wander on through our training areas, not chatting, each to our own world. In the rising warmth we turn into the gothic spires of a conifer plantation – tall, widely spaced trees allow shafts of sunlight to illuminate the nave. My eyes stretch to the sky, moving the forest round as I turn. It is so beautiful. The floor is a soft carpet of needles bouncing underfoot, windfall branches to make dens, four at least, some like a teepee, others in mid-air, tree branches masking their presence. There is a strong smell of pine, sweet and clean, cutting through the earthy loam lifting in the warming day. There are echoes of children's laughter, the shadows of small humans running through cloisters, mums and dads making homely additions to the dens, calling for Harry and Harriet to come and look.

Scout looks at me for a search command. I smile and tell him softly to go play, he gives my pocket a look, gets a treat and ambles off, me following, no rush, just slow time together. We've missed play in the last year; it feels a necessary luxury now.

He takes me to a fallen tree, large boulders tangled in grey roots, sweeping over the surface like rapids. He gives me the look and I see a small rock beautifully painted with a rainbow. I don't touch. There are more of these around now, people connecting with something elemental. Some people rage against them, but I don't mind the small offerings. Scout has found a feather, sniffing it from different angles, short intakes of scent, then a wait, his eyes glazing off into mid-space, then another sniff.

A flash on the edge of vision, something bright, colourful. A large dog bounds through the trees, its energy unnerving as it heads towards us, circles, then banks away. Scout stands and watches. I draw him closer. It has the look of a greyhound: blue marle coat, long legs and nose. A bright yellow jacket steps into a shaft of light. A woman holding the collar of a beautiful deerhound. I think about asking her to call the greyhound off but don't; it hasn't interfered with us, it's just enjoying pouring all its energy into this space. There are more dogs: two Border terriers on patrol, a dachs-hund weaving its way through all the obstacles, a brown Labrador that keeps waddling over to us, loses confidence and waddles away. It's a menagerie without any seeming rhyme or reason. I ask if they are all hers. The two sappers belong to old neighbours, the greyhound a nurse at work; it's crossed with a Border collie hence the blue marle. The deerhound is hers she says stroking its back – she's old and grumpy and not one for mixing. Scout lies at my feet, his nose sampling this motley crew.

The woman tells me when she first started coming to the forest, she could spend all day without seeing anyone, how wonderful it was to be free of the hum of life. Now she has to share it with people, few of whom stop to look at the beauty and listen to the centuries telling their tale. She laments the times we live now.

We part in thought, my feet attaching to a random path, Scout rooting around while I mull over the conversation with the yellow jacket. Why don't people spend more time looking, slowing down, appreciating what is around them? Mostly everyone seems to be in one great rush to get some-where else.

Scout finds another feather. It's clean, free of any woodland litter so must be new, an owl I think, the tan and white chevrons beautifully precise. How does nature do that? For all our technological know-how, humans still cannot do what nature can. The perfection of the feather pulls me into a moment transcending the smallness of human life – the world is vast, so much unknown. I wish I'd had more time when I was younger studying nature. I don't have regrets, I'm just more aware of the gaps in my education.

When I look up Scout's rock still, staring north. He shoots me a glance then returns to his watch. There is a steady warm breeze drifting down to us; I follow its direction and his gaze. At first, it's just trees, branches, a palette of light and shade that shimmers and shifts. As my eyes adjust the brain picks out shapes, something that should not be there; a deer and her fawn coalesce into focus. She's looking straight at us as we look back. The clocks have stopped. Above, thin cloud has ceased in motion. Time hangs. The fawn stays close to mum and does not look our way. Silence is heavy, the air thick with question, the smell of the woodland distilling into this space. Scout and I exchange a glance, then we both look back into the forest. It's empty. Where the deer and fawn were is now dappled light and shade. In their silence they have stepped back into their world taking something of us with them and leaving part of themselves within us.

At home Scout spends his days in ready observation, monitoring the movements of the household, his attention always on me.

He positions himself strategically around the house. Establishing observation posts at landings and hallways so that passage for myself and Alison is through a series of negotiated checkpoints. Each time I relocate requires the establishment of a new post, his body slumping down a wall on to the wooden floor with a gratifying thud, the air popping with the sound of smacking lips, sharp snorts punctuating the previously serene atmosphere. Once he is satisfied I am staying, he allows his body to slide to a prone position, chin resting on paws, everything orientated to me, a perfect line of sight, the whole performance culminating in a long audible sigh. Dotted around the house are smudges of grey wall where all else is bright clean white, and beneath, a floor buffed to a high sheen. If I manage to gain some moments of privacy behind a closed door, he lies across the threshold of the house – 'No one leaves this house but through me.' If we are in the same room his eyes track my every move, the whites waxing and waning as I cross his horizon. After settling he slips into a light snooze, the stillness and snoring stopping the instant he senses movement.

His inner clock announces mealtimes with unerring accuracy. He takes full advantage of his free movement around the house to initiate breakfast, surreptitiously edging the time forward, my day beginning five minutes earlier each morning until I reset his clock by locking the bedroom door for a Saturday lie-in.

Our morning routine begins with a cold wet nose tunnelled under blankets making contact with my warm sleeping skin, the shock bringing my consciousness abruptly into the world to see and hear two large black holes collecting night-time scents. Above the nose two eyes stare fixedly on mine. Once he has me out of bed he charges down to the kitchen, a bucket of nuts and bolts cascading down the wooden stairs ricocheting around the house and out into the street; his two older brothers frantically follow.

When I reach the kitchen, I find him fending off incursions from the others to the food store. Lips curled, teeth bared, nose scrunching up in mounting agitation, a growl rumbling to the surface from deep inside, his eyes alternating from food to the dogs as they probe the exclusion zone for any weakness. There are none.

As I fill bowls he switches to drool mode; great strands of super-gooey, slick saliva stream from his mouth, pooling across the floor like an incoming tide. This liquid is practically invisible, only apparent when a foot slides from under and a cry of shock and desperation ring out. Why no bones have been broken is perplexing.

Meals are taken in concentrated silence. The food consumed, each dog checks the food store and each other's bowls for any stray morsels, the steel bowls skating across the floor as tongues pick up the last speck of dust. Only when the store door is closed, and the bowls removed, does the room cease its spinning.

As the day's shadows lengthen Scout can be found outside the living room door like some alcoholic waiting for opening time. Once inside he claims his spot on the settee, stretched out full length, eyes drifting shut, pink tongue sticking out.

The day closes with a carrot, each dog scrabbling upstairs to consume in their night-time nests while we potter about. The Bedlingtons wallow down in soft beds; Scout seeks out his old armchair by the window, bathed in moonlight with a clear view of my sleeping form.

I listen to podcasts on long journeys – this feeds my latest obsession, the Appalachian Trail. This 2,200-mile US trail runs from Maine to Georgia and takes months to complete. I'd love to do something like this with Scout, closer to home. We have taken some multi-day walks and we have a new tent with plenty of room for both of us. He has his own mat and sleeping bag, his own PJs, and a backpack for snacks. It's wonderful walking with him; I can keep a conversation going with myself, not have to worry about boring him, or listen to his point of view. It's perfect.

We have a routine at camp. I pitch the tent, make the beds, then get on with a meal while Scout keeps a close watch. There is history here. As the food cooks he inches forwards until I move him away, then he stealth-creeps back one paw at a time. It's the only time our eyes never make contact – I reason he thinks if he can't see me then I can't see him. Like I say there's history. Once, I was cooking chunks of Spam, baked beans spiked with a little mustard, the aroma amazing, my stomach looking forward to the feast. Scout, his own food eaten, the bowl empty, sat transfixed, drool pouring out of his mouth. I turned, knocking the pan off the stove, the whole lot rolling across the grass. Not much I could do but let him have it all. I climbed into my sleeping bag hungry that night. Scout snuggled in his, happy, the tent pungent with his farts, snoring to keep the mountains awake, prayers offered to the god of dropped food.

We cruise through the narrow lanes, headlights sweeping the hedgerows, a flash of an owl on nocturnal forage, the sine wave of medieval hands ploughing the landscape. I like these nights, the summer day's warmth cloaking the soil, the moon pushing shadows across the fields.

Scout snoozes in the back, his bed warm from the heat of the city. A half hour back he'd stood in the kitchen watching as I checked my pack, running down the checklist – radio, head torch, map, clothing, food. When I take his coat off the peg, he knows we will be going to work. He'd been on the hill all day. Returned home to a dinner of biscuits and sardines, and whatever could be scrounged from the dinner plate and floor. After satisfying himself there was no more food he'd engaged the dishwasher pre-rinse cycle, then cleaned himself until the white gleamed and the black and tan framed his beauty. Then he rested. Keeping a clear view from the settee, down the hallway across the dining room into the kitchen to the fridge door and the cupboard where snacks are stored, and the door out of the house.

As we pull into the rendezvous, I note the handlers that have turned out. We're late, having the longest drive from the North, so we get what others have managed to dodge, usually ground that won't be easy to work, probably a lung-busting hill climb.

A white van stands in a pool of light; a thumping generator has cleared any roosting birds, and foxes that service the bins in the car park. A group of red jackets study maps and test radios, the huddle stepping back from the van's open door, thanking me for taking a leisurely drive over. I ask them if they need help finding their way out of the car park. They've been out for hours, the search expanding, reinforcements and more dogs arriving as night came. In the van a bearded man in heavy glasses and the aura of one who has seen it all before and would very much like to be home in a warm bed were it not for the fact someone somewhere needed help. He gives me the brief. A walking group paid a visit to the facilities in the car park, then carried on, returning to their car late afternoon, only realising when they notice the empty seat that one person is missing. The last time they can remember seeing the person was here. They think. I ask if I can speak to them, get an idea of the grey man. The beard shakes its head. They drove home after reporting him missing. With friends like that I say, he's better off lost. The beard nods. The thinking is he will have tried to make his way back to the car, got lost or suffered an injury. The only information we have is what his friends thought he was wearing; no one thought he had a map.

Scout is anxious to get going. I slip on his working coat, switch his light on and fix his bell. We have our little pre-game chat, telling him how much I love him, pressing my nose into the fur around his ears, nuzzling his snout with my cheeks then plastering him with kisses. He smells of warmth, and bed, and sleep. I promise him a trip to the seaside and a swim. His eyebrows bounce up and down.

There is access to our area through a private garden. Lights are on so I knock. A small woman, curlers, dressing gown, fluffy slippers, answers. I explain, apologise; the fluffy slippers look angry, so I play it low key, safe, ask about access through the garden. She spots Scout, shoves me out of the way to paw and coo over him, me standing redundant in the moonlight. She disappears inside, comes back with a digestive biscuit for Scout; he swallows it whole, I get nothing. There's lots of ear tweaking and forehead ruffling, Scout peering behind for another biscuit. Eventually, I manage to get the attention back on me, bringing a scowl from the fluffy slippers that shoo us out of the garden gate into our area. High-pitched squeals telling Scout what a lovely boy he is and how clever he is follow us until, thankfully, the darkness claims us. If the missing person is here, they must have heard that, I tell Scout.

The air is thick and heavy now the day has settled; heady wild garlic scent, a cacophony of fungi, blossom, and the earthy metallic smell of damp earth and cool limestone fill my senses. Monk's Dale sits in darkness for a moment until my eyes adjust. A stream runs down the centre, a path alongside strewn with limestone rubble. The air is still; we will have to take our time, work with thermal currents I can feel lifting from the water. The steep sides, thick with ivy and fallen trees will make it hard going.

We search small sections at a time working top to bottom to catch any human scent being lifted. We rest a minute at the end of each section, Scout getting a chunk of pemmican to keep his energy levels even.

Gradually we move through the landscape, back and forth across the stream; the further we penetrate the darker it becomes under the thick canopy. Occasionally we disturb an owl watching our progress, his voice floating a hole through the stillness. Scout ignores it. I can hear things scurrying below the fallen trees that have been left to provide a habitat for nature; fungi and mosses cover everything in tiny rainforests. Everything is life, decay and renewal.

After ninety minutes we take a rest by a wall where water bubbles up from the depths of the limestone world, the source of the stream, and right on point with the OS map. It's nice here in the silence of the night, a good spot for five minutes' rest, refuel and check the map.

As Scout works, I stay quiet and pay attention. If I feel an area needs searching more thoroughly I'll direct him with a word or an outstretched arm. Tonight, I encourage him up the steep side to a fence-line blocking anything but zealous progress beyond. If I see what looks like an entry into vegetation, called an 'in', often what humans think is a path, I run him along it until he can go no further. Many are rabbit runs and sheep tracks. I can hear him climbing near the fence, scrambling over tree trunks and thick ivy, his red light flashing in the darkness, the bell chiming.

Silence.

Everything has stopped. He's found something.

Emerging from the tangle of ivy he scans for me, finds me, then heads down. We've worked enough now for him to know that if he can see me, I can see him, and he can stay where he is and call me. Standing on a trunk he looks right at me and speaks, but he doesn't turn back to his find, he stays put. It means there isn't a body, but humans have been here recently. Another call, I start up the slope. It's tough going throwing legs over fallen trees, avoiding leg breakers, untangling limbs from ivy, and unhooking a pack from hanging branches. I'm sweating, my heart is pounding, my lungs complain.

Scout stands above monitoring my progress. The fence-line is rusty barbed wire, and a well-worn path. Far below I can see the silver ribbon of the stream in the moonlight and the first wisps of mist beginning to cloak the surface, the water glistening smooth and rich as it slides over cold, smooth limestone. I've climbed a hundred feet at a thirty-degree angle. Madness, just madness. Who in their right mind would be doing this in the early hours of a morning? Scout is sitting at the base of a tree, head proud, tail wagging. There is no stile, no gate, no footprints in the damp earth, only a trod in the undergrowth from below.

I ask Scout to show me; he barks, eyes swinging up the tree. I look for a pair of feet dangling. Nothing. Another look from Scout, something glistening in the crook of a branch. A bottle. This is what he's found; it must be recent to have human scent on. The label is new. Scout gets a reward while I work out what has happened. His nose must have caught scent settling down into the dale as the air has cooled; whoever left this, and their trail along the trod, has pulled him up to the tree. There's nowhere else to go from here so I'm certain it isn't our man. I mark the find on my map.

We move back down the slope, watching out for leg breakers, Scout skipping from one fallen trunk to another. Scout drinks long and slow from the cold spring, quenching his thirst and clearing his olfactory chambers.

The dale opens out; Scout takes the opportunity to stretch his legs, releasing the tightness from the last hours. A layer of fine mist is suspended above the meadow; gossamer wisps pulled and twisted by his movement swirl languorously. We've worked for four hours to clear Monk's Dale. Now we are out of the towering sides of the dale I have radio communication. We're told to stand down. It's a good outcome. The police have located the grey man tucked up in bed at home, unaware he had been reported missing. After finding his friends gone, he'd made his way to the cars to find those gone too. So, he'd made his way home. We'll be picked up by a team vehicle in a little while.

There's a bench by the road where we unpack our food and rest. Scout watches closely, his eyes and nose following his filled bowl as it arcs to the ground. I pour tea and bite into the sandwich Alison made. Preparation for a call-out is now well choreographed at home. I get dressed, make any calls, pick up my pack, and, as I step out of the door, Alison hands me flask, sandwich, nibbles and treats for his lordship. Tonight, it's cheese and harissa on sourdough, a flask of Assam, a bag of crisps, an apple for my health. Scout has kibble, pemmican. No Tunnock's.

It's 4 a.m. and we're heading home as the world lifts from sleep. On the horizon the deep indigo of night has split into a pink and grey bank of daybreak; inversions are building in the long valleys leaving islands of rock to meet the rising dawn.

Scout, snuggled up in his bed, snores deeply in contentment.

Sitting to the north of Leek just within the Peak District National Park, the hill of Gun is a good vantage point over the vast plain that stretches out to the west coast. In the centre sits a flat gleaming white dish pointing at worlds unknown to me, the result of Bernard Lovell messing around in a field with army surplus kit. Jodrell Bank.

We went once, Alison and I. A beautiful summer's day, happened upon it by chance as we scooted along thin roads, wandered in. It had low flat-roofed prefabs, paths, lawns, a look of dignified academic neglect cradling the engineering marvel. I spent a happy hour tracing the filigree steelwork, straining to see if I could hear crackles and pops, remembering those child-hood black-and-white sci-fi films. We sat on the lawn drinking tea from the funny works canteen, watching a man on a roof in a beige cardigan, brown striped shirt with a big collar, seventies, ginger straggly beard. A sign said *Flat Roof, Caution*. No one paid him any attention, people sat, drank, ate cake, discussed what they would have for tea – ham or chicken, with salad, and a trifle. Tomorrow cut the grass.

The air swam with whistles and pops from the enormous speaker on the roof. The man's voice mingled with the sound, the voice cultured, intelli-gent, trying to hold down its excitement as it worked toward the big reveal. That sound, he said, comes from a star billions of light years from Earth. He took us on an auditory journey through the universe and beyond, the great dish swinging across the sky searching for a find. We sat and listened with eyes closed, lost to the cosmos as the stream of data swirled around us. It didn't matter we didn't know what it meant. For a brief period of time, we crossed into another place.

The dish still looks beautiful today, the resonance passing through as I sit on Gun. To the west sits The Cloud where the summer solstice sun will set, rise, and set again. Beyond The Cloud, the mountains of Wales. To the north, the silt layers from the age before time, the gritstone edges of The Roaches, Hen Cloud. To the south, the hills of Houseman, of a generation lost, their remnants lying in the soil. And beyond, the Brecon Beacons, brooding, crouching down into the landscape, their flanks turned against the inter-minable wind and rain. East the Fenlands and the North Sea. And here Gun, the centre of all.

I find a shallow bowl of heather and bilberry to hunker down from the westerly, cold for the time of year. The petrol station cheese and egg sand-wich washed down with tepid bitter iced coffee does not lift my spirits. I am here to scope out a walk for my next guidebook. This morning had been gentle and long, the easy gradient letting my body rest and my mind wander. I felt the loneliness.

I left Scout at home, something I had dithered about for days. On our last walk, there'd been inquisitive cows. And an attack on Scout from a farm dog had left him shaken. He'd shown some hesitancy in training after; I suspected he still had some trauma. Fearful there might be a repeat, too many farms on the map, I decided to come on my own. But there are few cows and fewer farm dogs. I feel sad and guilty he is not with me. I am surprised how much I miss his company, how big the space where he should have lain by me in the heather and bilberry is.

No longer under assessment, I had relaxed and passed that down the leash. Out walking, Scout explored ahead until we stopped for a break when he'd sit on his haunches watching me pull food and drink out of my pack. The fresh water he ignored, preferring a fly-strewn muddy hoof print. Once finished with his food, he'd turn attention to mine using mind games and saliva, my mind pummelled by waves of energy, my trousers soaked with drool. Having exhausted supplies, he would settle, the eyelids gradually falling, the tongue poking out.

Today, I am alone. The feeling of separation is new and unpleasant. Once, when I was without him due to his injury, someone said I must be pleased I didn't have him with me. I thought no, I'd sooner be with Scout than with you. I'd thought about that a lot. Never walked without him again. I used to think the best number of people for walking is one. Now I add a dog.

What will it be like when he is gone? I headed for home, walking those thoughts out of my head. Of late I've felt something deeper that, as yet, I have no understanding of. More than words. There is an emotional current flowing between us that I cannot quite fathom. When did we become so bound to each other?

That evening, I sit with Scout stroking him. Perhaps all he asks is that I keep my side of the contract – be faithful, be protective, be loving – as he does with me.

As summer drifts into autumn our days are filled with walking, writing, cooking and eating. Sundays are for training in the valley; Thursday evenings we train in the forest, on the Common or Wharncliffe Chase on the edge of the forest, with its rocky edges, long open spaces and heath. With Paul, Annette and Diane we can mix and match scenarios to hone our skills. We get a new face one night, the poet Helen Mort. Helen is an old friend of Scout; he'd modelled for the cover of her book *Never Leave the Dog Behind*. Now, when I walk into a bookshop, I see Scout looking out from a shelf.

This had started his modelling career. He's been the centrepiece for a double-page spread in a national outdoor magazine, about mountain rescue search dogs. Completed an advertising assignment for bacon on Staithes beach, a dream job. People snatch selfies with him. A dogsbody has a photo, with Scout looking into her eyes, on her bedside table.

I've completed the guidebook. Scout accompanying me on most of the walks, up to thirty kilometres a day, Scout doing at least double. It's honed his body, which has grown lithe and supple, his limbs strong, his body cinched at the waist, allowing his powerful haunches to articulate with easy, graceful movement over rock and moor. He never tires, never complains, just keeps going to the end.

The last few autumns Alison has been teaching at the university's campus in Wuhan, China. This meant me and the dogs were home alone for several weeks, which meant meat. Alison, being a vegetarian, pretty much made me one at home. The local butchers loved it, as did the dogs, and they promised not to tell. As soon as her plane left the ground I'd be down at the butcher with a list, he'd nod knowingly, wrapping steaks, sausages, chops, give me a wink and whisper out of the corner of his mouth, 'Seein' as the wife's away I've put a little something extra in.' The shiny dark brown liver would be looking up at me as I unwrapped the parcel, a note scribbled on the paper: *mum's the word*. The dogs crowded me as I packed the meats into the fridge, each pushing to be in front.

Alison isn't going this year. The last visit she'd been seriously ill with a chest infection; it left her gasping for breath and drained of energy, and the last twelve months taking some powerful drugs for a respiratory disease. It was a worrying time. Even though she's had the 'all clear' her energy levels can still be low. She took early retirement, so we see more of each other now and the dogs get long walks and rest while Alison meditates in her favourite forest clearing.

Because of our skill and experience, we are called to search for despondent and vulnerable people who have reached a point where living is no longer an option. Often the edgelands, those liminal spaces between road and rail along the outskirts of towns, the post-industrial sites long abandoned to nettle and rosebay willowherb, wasteland turned into nature reserves. One dog has a find a few metres from a path in a country park, people strolling, the missing person finally free of life. We search golf courses at all hours. I'm not a fan of golf or golfers, those strange-looking clothes, but they leave us alone to get on with the work and I keep Scout away from the greens. He ignores all the lost balls he finds – I promise him one night we will return and make our fortune. We search the edges of housing, checking old dens, climbing over stained mattresses, rusting white goods, nettles springing out of shiny washing machine drums. We search alongside the police. One weekend we search a lakeside, the police on the other side of the hedge. Scout comes back and indicates, takes me through a hole in the bushes to a terrified group of youths frantically wafting away the stench of weed. I mention the place is crawling with police and they exit like a split atom.

On a morning of torrential rain, we search a nature reserve for a despondent person, who'd left behind a message, keys and mobile phone. It's an old industrial site, quiet, out of the way. The perfect spot for a few last moments of peace. The rain bounces off bushes as we work around the various ponds. Police and team sections are also out; we eject six policewomen ambling through our area chatting to each other. The search controller radios to say the missing person has been found in a bird hide sleeping off last night's excess. The rain has stopped.

I realise this is the scrapyard that fed the melting shop where I worked in the 1980s. I can see the huge building through the bushes, anchored like a great liner from a bygone age. It's a theme park now, teaching children what work used to be like. I can see where I cut down old steam pipes that ran the length of the building, tearing asbestos off to get at the metal so we could burn it through with oxy torches, twenty feet of steel falling to the ground. Then walking a new bigger pipe up the ladder, dead weight digging into shoulders, knees taking the strain, the ladder curving into the wall, slipping an inch or two, but you kept going. The weather was glorious that summer; we were happy to be outside and even happier to sink pints of beer at the end of the shift, even if you were scratching from all the asbestos that had floated through the air. The pipe is still there, unused now.

They were good days with good people. We were set for life with the security of a key industry. In the early 1970s no one had heard of trickle down, privatisation, Thatcherism. Back then we had society. By 1985 it would all be over, steel and coal gone, redundancy spent on buying the council house, a new front door, a week in Benidorm and a new Datsun Sunny. I got a job selling pipefittings, driving round the country in an Austin Montego, the worst car ever made.

Dad died in 1981, riddled with cancer. Me and Mum looked after him. Dad didn't know what was wrong with him or that he was dying, he thought he had varicose veins. Mum forbade any talk of it, not to Dad, or anyone else, definitely not to neighbours. At first, I thought it was to protect Dad, only later did I realise she didn't want the street to know we had trouble. Death had crept up the street, taking mostly men, but some women, people who had worked in steel, coal, construction. Now it was our turn.

The lads at work protected me through Dad's illness; word had got out. I'd been moved on to a day shift so I could give Mum a break at night. I'd come home early afternoon and sit with Dad, chat, sometimes in the garden when the weather was fine, sometimes when he was in bed, the disease overwhelming him. One day I found him on the settee worrying about getting back to work, not having money, being thrown out of the council house. I could see then what life had done to him, made him afraid, how scared he had been. He broke down and sobbed, his face in gnarled hands, the thin bony shoulders hardly registering movement. I held him in my arms, told him all would be well, that I'd take care of us, kissed his head and felt him lean into me. I held him for a long time, till the sobbing ceased. I walked for hours in the woods that night though I don't remember the trees.

As his end drew near, I'd sleep by his bed, Mum in my room to give her some rest. Dad got it into his head to get downstairs. I knew if he did, we'd never get him back up to the bedroom. I'd stop him, settle him back beneath the blankets, only to hear him rise again with a need for the toilet. I'd take him, clean him up, then he'd make a clumsy, stumbling dash, the pyjamas falling around wasted legs while we waltzed on the landing, him shouting in his thin rasping voice, Mum coming out all flustered. We'd finally get him back to bed and I'd stare at the ceiling until the walls became light.

I pushed all this well away from me – didn't think, went to work, ignored the pain at home, the steelworks becoming a sanctuary for me. Dad died in the summer, helped on his way by a Brompton Cocktail. I never got the chance to say thank you, I love you, goodbye. I think of him every day, how much he gave and how much he never had. I miss him.

After that, the family disintegrated, that atom again, smashed to all corners. My brother got married; it didn't last. I bought a house, picked up where I'd left off with the booze. Somewhere in the midst of it all, got married, got divorced. It wasn't a pleasant experience for anyone. I put the drink down in 1988, found people who could help me, who I could trust. Many are still around today; we are all still sober. The mental stuff was more problematic, not helped by being unable to handle rejection. After two decades of running at the same wall, and being successful, I threw in the towel and began the life I have today with Alison. She was the key that unlocked the world I always wanted. It isn't possessions or title or even a job for life.

The real wealth of happiness and contentment stemmed from our first date – I just followed that new thread.

Mum died a few years back, thirty-three years after Dad; she was the last of the neighbours to go. She died peacefully in the same council house Dad worried about losing. Most of his years my brother has lived there too. The furnishings haven't changed, the decorating last done by Dad. Dad's wallpaper now held up with bits of Sellotape.

Sobriety and Alison gave me the courage to step out into a new life and I began exploring the remote mountain landscape of Britain. On Valentine's Day in thick snow and strong winds I stepped across a small brook; my mind still sees my crampon boot sinking into the snow. Thirty minutes later I came to, lying in snow surrounded by boulders. I passed out several times. I remember a dog, a hand gently holding me down and a voice saying I was safe. I went back in summer, trying to piece together what happened. To this day I guess only the raven knows. A year later I joined mountain rescue.

I've seen thousands get sober and build a good life, find happiness. And I've known hundreds stick with drink and die by their own hand. I feel for those that want to exit life, but I feel more for those they leave behind, who will always have questions, always wonder if they were responsible.

I've noticed there is a difference in what is left behind when we find a deceased person. Perhaps I'm sensitive to this, maybe it's my imagination. The unplanned death seems to leave the person's soul – being, call it what you will – with the physical body, as though there wasn't enough time to prepare. Someone who has taken their own life leaves a sense that whatever spoke of their human spirit has left; all we see is the vessel that carried the life. It's as though the person, the one who laughed and smiled and told people they loved them, and when asked said they were fine, had finally gained release.

October brings a call-out to Loxley Common. We're there first. I send Scout off to find the casualty in the labyrinth of paths and covering of trees, even though we have a location. I'm fully expecting it to be a dog walker I know, probably someone we saw this morning. He comes back to tell me he has found them and gets his reward as the little group of people look on in bemusement, wondering why mountain rescue has turned up to play ball with a dog. After his reward I explain and go back to the rendezvous to guide those following. A casualty with a busted knee got treatment a little bit quicker because Scout did his job.

A walker-cum-wild camper – no map or torch, just a phone – has become benighted high on Bleaklow. Nerves had taken over as the dark enveloped and their world shrunk. Rather than set up the tent and bunker down till morning they've called for help. The police think it's a remote spot over rough ground and call the team. We get a phone lock on the person's position and instruct the walker to stay there and wait. Experience says the person will move, eager to show they are not completely without ability. A couple of police constables stand by watching the team getting ready to deploy, while a snatch squad of fell runners set off in a Land Rover up a shooting track to yomp across the moor to the location. We get ready without any rush – it's a fine night with weather on our side, there's no need for heroes. Scout and I, plus a navigator, are tasked with walking up to a ridge to block any escape routes the person might try. The police leave as we discuss a route; a few kilometres up a gently rising moor will keep us out of the deep groughs and bogs.

We've been on the hill for about thirty minutes when Scout sets off into the wind, his form disappearing over a slight rise, his bell and light telling me where he is. There is a deep grough in that area, one of a series that are exhausting to cross – it's why we're taking a circuitous route. Scout comes back to tell me he's found. Surely not, perhaps it's someone out for a bivvy. Scout leads us to two figures standing on the edge of the grough looking in. They're dressed in hi-vis jackets, black trousers, safety shoes. Probably a couple of lads that have been watching too many wild camping videos on YouTube. Both are shining phones into the depths of the grough, the light disintegrating in less than a metre. It's the two police constables from the rendezvous.

'What are you two doing?'

'Going to get the casualty.'

'Does anyone know you are here?'

'No. We had to come because you lot were fucking about.'

The male shows me a Google map, shoving the phone at me with the lost person's location marked with a pin. It's a kilometre and half away, the map just a pleasant light green. No crags, no groughs, no water courses, no featureless moor, no hills or valleys, all of which will need to be crossed on their trajectory.

I am far from happy, especially with the last comment.

'You need to fuck off back to the road.' I sense my navigator take a step closer.

'You can't talk to us like that, we're the police.'

'I don't give a fuck who you are, you're interfering with a call-out. Fuck off. Now.'

They turn away and look back down the grough, their first obstacle, and they're defeated. They're a liability on the hill and interfering with an operation. If the walker really was down there, the police scent might mask the person's presence, cause an unnecessary distraction, contaminate the ground for Scout. I need them off the hill. I radio our search manager and ask him to contact the police to get their two wannabe heroes off the moor before they become another casualty.

My navigator stands open-mouthed. Scout stands in disbelief having not had a reward for his find. I give him a few minutes' play while I make sure the two constables plod off the moor in defeat.

The benighted walker is found. We take a gentle amble back across the moor to the rendezvous. It's a beautiful night, the air crystal clear, the lights of the north twinkling around us. Back at the control van the police have gone.

Snow arrives in November giving us hours of fun on the high moors and crags. It's a glorious landscape of thick undisturbed powder and deep drifts laid out beneath blue skies. We have snowball fights, me showing Scout one I've made then tossing it into a drift, Scout diving in head first trying to find it, surfacing with little hills of snow all over his head, a snowflake on the tip of his nose, me aching with joy and love. I manage to get shots of walkers and runners for magazine articles and – to my delight – a climber ascending Alport Tower. It's set in the deep, long Alport Dale that took the lives of those youths in 1964. Today, it's a picture of beauty and serenity, the climber adding the final touch to the landscape. Scout has his socks and boots on to stop snow packing his toes with ice. I hide treats in the snow for him and he tunnels away, beaming a great smile as he surfaces with the treasure. It's a great time to live, how I had always dreamed our winter days to be: white powder, blue sky, Scout enjoying every minute. I am happy, truly happy.

I take my winter fitness tests, Cut Gate in sixty-five minutes, Parkin Clough in twenty-six. Slower than last year, Parkin Clough harder. I've just clicked past sixty years old and feel good if a little on the heavy side – hills have me panting a little more, my legs pleading for more oxygen. Lose weight, put in some jogging and I'll be fit for the upgrade assessment in two years.

We get flu jabs now though I still get a few chest infections, the last few hanging around for months.

As the year closes, we've become operational after three years of training; Scout has attended numerous call-outs, we've put in 600 hours of mountain rescue time, located a casualty, two plodding wannabe heroes, and a fledgling teen drug cartel. We've had a good year.

2020

The first day of the new decade and a walker is lost on Kinder Scout. We make our way through dull roads in grey weather, the prospect of hours searching the deep groughs and barren moor only inviting for Scout who is happy to be out. We are stood down on our way through the back roads to the rendezvous, the walker found by another and guided to safety. We turn for home to finish the last of the Christmas pudding and cream, and chocolates, a New Year's resolution not surviving past midnight on the first day.

The country is still mired in Brexit. Following on from austerity, the impact on people's well-being is becoming more evident. The weft and warp of our communities slowly being pulled to breaking point as those in need are shoved further from the centre, the disparity between the haves and havenots expanding at an alarming rate. One side poor health, low wages, poor education, fewer opportunities; the other side wealthy, well educated, connected, a life full of opportunities – often there is only a few miles between those two sections of society, the fortunate living a decade or more longer. Everything seems to be about money; the car a symbol of how successful you are and therefore what kind of person you are or want to be seen as. The news is filled with politicians shouting about immigration, and the sunlit uplands leaving the European Union has released. But many feel they have less of everything – less money, less influence, less importance.

The impact on mountain rescue is a regrouping of some members along political lines. On the whole, people get on with each other, most teams have a small-c conservatism, with the odd person way out on the right, some left-leaning members, with the odd one outlying. Brexit creates a few arguments, some falling out with long-term friends. As I'm very much on the left, with a belief in a fairer society, I'm already tagged a communist and called 'Red'.

Since Brexit, I've been getting emails from Conservative Campaign Headquarters. I know exactly who is responsible for signing me up to the Conservative Party, the only problem is that I don't have the password to cancel the membership. I make the appropriate noise as handlers hide smiles.

As temperatures drop, snow lays another blanket on the landscape and Scout and I head to Bamford Edge. We head up a hollow way through ancient woodland; twisted branches add a fairytale feel. He gets a scent and strikes. I trudge after him, slower than usual, the sharp cold pinching my lungs. I take a sharp intake to inflate my chest until I get the satisfactory popping, the restriction giving way. Maybe it's the ribs damaged in the fall I had? The air rushes in and I feel the oxygen flowing into muscle. I'm getting this feeling more – the lungs popping outwards – and I always make a pact to lose weight, Alison supporting my efforts with healthy eating. Fewer clandestine visits to KFC and McDonald's might also help. Scout comes tearing round the corner and skids to a halt against my boots, barks, then spins away. He's found.

There is no body, just empty yellow packets of biscuits, empty Coke bottles. Scout digs out booty, wolfing down a pork pie he's sniffed out under the snow. I remember the spot. Last summer finding a young man here when we were out walking. He'd bags of shopping and was well out of the way. He was nervous. I got the sense he didn't want to be found and I'd asked him if he was okay. He'd nodded, shifted the weight from one foot to the other, remained silent. We'd left him to his summer retreat, I'd kept an eye on social media for a missing person but saw nothing, and as months slipped by, he'd gone from my mind. Until Scout found the site. Now there are just my footprints and Scout's.

On a fine winter night, we thread through Pennine mill towns to search for a despondent person, their car found near a reservoir, a note left at home for a family wringing their hands past the hour of sleep. We search inbye fields, old farms, some derelict, some turned into desirable residences with big plate windows, cobbled drives and fancy gates. There's a full moon and good light, clouds scudding shadows across the land, trees as black as charcoal rattling as the wind whistles through. A thousand eyes stare back as I sweep my headtorch by. It takes me a while to register I was here last year researching a guidebook walk. I like the South Pennines, it is still a living landscape. Having escaped the clutches of the national park lobby, its communities have continued to be vibrant and alive with culture, art and local food playing central roles.

A trail dog has tracked the missing person's scent to a gate leading on to a high moor, then lost the trail. The dog and handler aren't trained for moorland work – this is tough terrain, so we are tasked to search. It's square miles of featureless peat and grass. We find nothing. Later that day police divers find the missing person sat at the bottom of the reservoir with a car battery. The theory is, they left the car, walked up to the gate for a view of the setting sun, then returned, picked up the battery and walked into the water.

The team takes time to pick up traction in training, all those mince pies dragging the legs. We have a night exercise coming up; I discuss it with Steve. We've both had poor experiences when other people set up an exercise with dogs. If there is anyone that knows how to set up a search exercise it's a dog handler, but we are rarely consulted. I set our own exercise up within the team's, leaving a rucksack earlier that day on a high contour in the hope that a Good Samaritan doesn't come across it and hand it in, though I stick a note to the outside just in case. It has my clothing and it's hidden tight against a wall on the upwind side. We will approach from downwind. With the wall in the way of the flow, I want to see how far we get before Scout detects the scent. We'll find the team casualty first as part of the overarching exercise then leave for our own jaunt.

It's cold and clear, a full moon, hares dart away as we get near, sheep loom out of the darkness. The wind is running straight down the moor from the cache I've set. We find the team casualty first, leaving quickly so foot search sections do not see the location. It's a steep rise on to the moor, the wind blowing above our heads as we climb in the lee. Scout makes easy progress showing no signs of scent until we crest the hillside to meet the wind barrelling into our faces. It triggers him immediately, pulling away from me for the scent dump 600 metres away. I figure the wall is acting as a weir, rolling the wind over the top and leaving a dead zone at the base downwind. I'm expecting the scent cone to disappear as Scout gets to the wall; I want to see what he does. When he gets there, sure enough the scent is diminished. He roots around the base until he picks up some crumbs, follows them up the wall and hops on top. He's worked it out. He drops down then back on top like a jack-in-the-box to tell me he has found and hurry up.

Lately, he's started telling me he's found when he can see me, rather than returning, being impatient with my slow progress. Our roles are reversing, as our fitness levels converge then cross. He's almost four now, feeling his body can do anything. He's growing into a commanding dog and stepping up in charge.

We finish with a saunter back under the full moon. It's good to get out, breathe some fresh air and release tension. There's anxiety around the country; people fleeing war and famine fill news bulletins and fuel fears of the country being overrun. In China, a virus is causing problems around Wuhan; I wonder if this is what Alison suffered from on her final visit. The prime minister says he's been shaking hands with abandon. There is nothing to be afraid of.

The next national training weekend is in the Peak District and I'm setting up areas around the crags and moorland of Burbage Moor. It's a busy day – a fell race passing through, an orienteering competition criss-crossing our area, lots of people with bikes and dogs. Children scatter on to boulders – superhero stuff – while actual climbers dangle from ropes along the crag. It will be interesting to see how the dogs and handlers cope with all this. I watch bodies going into position; the other handlers are back in the car park to keep the exercise blind. Scout stands by me on a boulder mesmerised by all that is flowing this way and that.

Something pulls my jacket. I look down to see a small boy with a runner's number covering most of his body. He's wearing a T-shirt and shorts; it's around zero degrees in the sun. He tells me he's lost his dad. He's anxious and he's shivering. I bury him in my jacket and radio for hot tea and some biscuits, then sit him on Scout's boulder who closes into the lad adding his body warmth to the spindly red legs. He gives Scout cuddles, drinks warm tea and is forced to share his digestives with Scout. I think we'll keep him here while we get in touch with his dad. I ask if he wants to continue. A shrug while he feeds Scout another biscuit. He seems happy enough, Scout certainly is. 'I'll phone the race controller to come and pick you up.' I get a smile, a nod, Scout gets another biscuit. The handler who'd been looking forward to the biscuits looks more depressed at each passing digestive. He digs out a Mars bar from his pack. It must have been there for a few years as an emergency ration – it's mangled and hard with bits of gooey stuff and fluff stuck to the wrapper. Now the lad and Scout look sad. A mother appears full of thanks; the boy is gathered into her arms. The lad had done well, done the right thing, we say. Scout stares at the handler holding what remains of the biscuits.

A shadow just out of vision seeps into the nation's subconscious. It picks at warning bells just enough to hold a thought that something is not right.

The cessation of normal life comes quickly. It has a name: Lockdown. It turns out that the Chinese virus, as they call it, from Wuhan, and of no consequence to the West, is of great consequence. Tens of thousands are dying around the world, their lungs filling with fluid leaving them fighting for every single tiny breath until they cease the fight and join others piled high in mortuaries, leisure centres and meat freezers. In the UK it begins, as it does in every other country, with one or two isolated cases. Each day the numbers climb ever higher – those infected, those dead – a macabre TV game to see if the nation can hit 10,000 deaths, 100,000 deaths, half a million?

Everything stops. No planes, trains or cars. No work, no shops, no factories, no offices. Only those who can treat people work: the front line, the only line. No one mixes. Birthdays, weddings, funerals all cancelled. Families separated from each other. Students incarcerated in halls of residence. Food can be bought; individuals queue to walk around dystopian supermarkets keeping a minimum two-metre distance, avoiding contact, avoiding words, avoiding looking. Toilet rolls and antibacterial hand cleanser which kills 99.9 per cent of everything have to be rationed; fights break out for the last roll and bottle. If hand cleanser kills just about everything, why not just take a swig of it? Some do. Tin foil hats are next; conspiracists crank up the volume. Websites crash with requests for deliveries of food, booze and fags. No one has a face mask; the world scrambles for supplies. It is a gold mine for some. An allowance of a daily walk of indeterminate length for an unspecified period of time is allowed. Other than that, stay indoors. Each night we watch the telly: men in suits – politicians, doctors – stand clutching lecterns telling us how bad it is and how bad it is going to get. Nurses and doctors have purple and black imprints of goggles and masks etched on to their faces. We clap for them at 8 p.m. each Thursday, stand in the street and clap. Someone plays 'Somewhere Over the Rainbow' on a flute; we clap again, see who is still around, turn back into the house, close the door, make tea. Covid has arrived.

• • •

With restrictions on movement and no work, soon the well-known paths are exhausted, and new ones are found. Courtesy becomes normal; people step aside to allow others to pass. Passing places emerge; no one wants to be infected. We see the ventilators on the news, the large plastic tubes down throats. It is that we fear most, not the virus.

The first week, Alison's father dies, old age. In hindsight a blessing; at ninety-three he probably would not have made it. Lockdown means she cannot attend, there's no funeral. It will be two years before she receives his ashes.

After the first few days, the air is crystal clear, the city becomes sharp and vivid, the horizon has moved so far back the sea can be seen. You can feel how clean everything is. This is a new way of life, away from making money for others; there is an alternative. We've been lied to. The aroma of home-made bread fills streets, social media is awash with how to live differently, man caves are constructed at the bottoms of gardens, builders' merchants struggle with demand. The cities begin emptying. The fortunate few move to the country, a slower pace of life, away from the virus. National parks change from being 'Yours' to 'Ours' – they no longer belong to all of us. Vociferous in telling visitors to stay away from their communities, hand-painted boards appear on major routes, shouting *Stay Home*. Police drones hunt down walkers on gritstone edges; motorcyclists are fined.

Words pop up: hygge, sourdough, repair, knitting, sewing, drawing, natural fibres, van life. The big thing on the internet is how-to videos about alternative lifestyles, Scandi log cabins, rundown wrecks on Italian mountains, converting an old Transit van into a luxury mobile home. Online masterclasses in everything proliferate. Celebrities share pearls of wisdom. People clutch at anything, trying to make sense of it all.

Children's playgrounds are sealed with hi-vis tape, the swings chained high above; wooden pallets block slides. Local golf courses, without fanfare, quietly open their fairways for people to walk; no one walks on the greens. In the city, deer appear in the concrete canyons as nature claims back the spaces we have taken away. One swims upriver to the forest, the human landscape holding nothing for wildlife. The number of dead keeps rising.

As the country settles into a daily groove of exercise and yet more bread, those who have never really walked before, young and old, succumb to injury. Every team in the country sees a massive increase in call-outs creating a singularly unique problem: how to keep team members, dogs and the casualty safe from infection. We wear full protection – face masks, goggles, gloves, zipped-up jackets – hardly an inch of skin showing, the team split into sections to avoid cross-contamination. It's mainly adults we rescue – broken ankles, popped knees, dislocated shoulders. Unused to the terrain, the unevenness underfoot, old bone and sinew unable to balance the ungainly mass. We pick them up, carry them miles on a stretcher; in the heat of summer it's unpleasant, but who else is there to do it? The same members attend, those without family and children. After a call-out everything has to be decontaminated, adding hours to the day, because no one is sure how the virus spreads. I keep Scout away from other dogs and people, in case his coat can carry it from someone stroking him. Operating largely unseen, we strive to end each day in one piece. No one claps for mountain rescue.

In the summer, infection and death rates fall, restrictions are relaxed. No one is prepared for what happens as the starting gun is fired: everyone heads for the hills. People now released want the life they have seen on YouTube, the life they have dreamed of. Vans clog lay-bys. Humans swarm across the countryside, away from infected cities where hospitals are full. Human waste and litter quilt the land. Locals get angry. People venture into more remote areas, many with little or no experience. In just a few months mountain rescue teams exceed the annual number of call-outs, a mixture of low experience and lack of hill fitness, or inexperienced and overwhelmed by terrain and conditions, or just plain lost.

Social media has perfect images of camping by perfect lakes or a perfect view from a mountain top, or those perfect hidden places. Nothing is unachievable.

On a windy night search for two frightened campers, we come across twenty tents on Kinder Scout, the occupants of each one woken to ask if they had called for help. Having seen videos of a fell runner dancing through a remote Peak District wilderness, a novice runner is overwhelmed by conditions during a major storm around Laddow Rocks and calls for help, triggering a major search operation with several teams and dogs. For six hours we search in horrendous weather, Scout clearing Wessenden Head Moor, Steve and his dog Moss clearing Black Hill, while foot sections cleared main paths. Each time the missing person called, they had moved location again. The search would swing around, only to find the spot empty. The Coastguard helicopter arrived in the early hours of the morning. Police made further enquiries as the weather deteriorated and concern for life increased. In the hour before dawn, in our third search area, wet and covered in dark peat from numerous bogs, we are stood down. The missing person found at home, having not thought to tell anyone they were safe, but complaining bitterly the hills should not be open in such weather.

In another part of the country a team member suffers significant injuries and subsequently dies after being called to rescue two campers.

A party, one with a broken leg, call for help. Having eventually found a phone signal they give a location from a smartphone app, then go back to the broken leg, a few hundred metres away, not realising that their location has now moved. When the team arrives, the location is bare. Scout is deployed and finds them in the trees, helping the casualty before a long wait for an ambulance.

No matter how many pleas are made for people to think and be careful, people have a need for release. Mountain rescue always respond.

At the end of lockdown, many suffering from mental health and well-being issues – isolated, a support system already eroded by austerity and further crippled by a pandemic – seek release. Reservoirs are favoured, woodland, the remote and secluded. Drownings, hangings, self-harm, drugs and alcohol. Whatever the circumstances they have to be found. For the dogs what matters is the finding of a human, leading to their reward. It is the handler and navigator who attend to those who have found their release. In time, more team members arrive, and the police to complete their own tasks. Then the body removed to a waiting vehicle, the place cloaked in silent respect.

The price is heavy in many quarters. The pandemic has seen the number of suicides the team attend increase greatly. It leaves an imprint on team members, and they need to decompress, to work through thoughts and emotions, feel their feet on firm ground again. In time, some leave, unable to hold the experience in their normal daily life any longer. For some, the boundary into mental illness is crossed, post-traumatic stress threads through the days, people ostracise and are ostracised, friendships are broken, and made.

There is a vein that runs through mountain rescue, it's about manliness, and being tough, of not succumbing. It can help – extreme weather calls for resilience and a toughness. But it can mean that those in trouble with mental health and emotional issues can become isolated, fearful of being seen as weak. And in a tiny minority of cases, vulnerability is seen as weakness by those too immature to see it as someone needing help, and, like a pack of hyenas, someone's ego will attack those they see as weaker. Few people talk about mental health, bullying can often be prevalent in such cases, and being volunteers there is little support. For some, the pandemic will exacerbate an already unstable mindset, and they will also seek release. It is a huge price to pay.

We take the opportunity for a holiday and hire a cottage on the Pembrokeshire coast for a week of summer sun. I'm tired, and on edge, prone to flare-ups of anger at the slightest thing. Alison treads on seashells while the dogs keep out of my way. After a few days I manage to bring myself down. My mood is not helped by the cough that seems to be a permanent fixture. Several in the team have complained about coughs and chest infections, unable to shake them off completely. We put it down to having to wear masks for long periods of time while breathing heavily as we carry a stretcher. At the beach, the warmth of the sun, the expanse of sand and sea draw me out of myself. Alison smiles, suggests a swim as she runs off with the dogs, Scout tearing in front for a full-body launch into the waves. I saunter down hoping it won't be too cold. It is. Alison is already in, coaxing little Monty deeper. It's not his favourite pastime; he shows willingness but soon steers a course for the shore, shakes himself, then looks with contempt at the others. I pull long strokes into deeper water. I'm a strong swimmer; Dad taught me well on our annual holiday in Blackpool.

It's a memory I cherish, a happy time. Dad encouraging me, telling me how well I was doing, the saltiness filling my mouth making me cough and splutter, the greenness of the sea, the waves splashing up the pier legs. He'd get me to go a little deeper but keep me safe, never taking me beyond my limit. I was so happy at having his approval, of pleasing him. We swam together, side by side, his face happy and smiling. There in that mucky water amidst the smell of hot dogs and chips, the sound of fairground rides and crashing waves, I had the best dad in the world.

Scout swims breaststroke, not doggy-paddle, his strong limbs powering through the water drawing long arcs, his body at ease, loving the waves so much. Over the next few days he teaches himself to surf. He works out that in the shallows the waves are too small, spent of energy, there's no feeling of weightlessness. He swims through these, to the bigger surf that rolls ahead. By trial and error, he finds the perfect wave that lifts him free of gravity for a few glorious moments. I watch him relish the feeling of floating to the beach high on the surf, a broad smile on his face. He heads straight back in. Crowds gather to watch. He plays the audience, and I have a hard time getting him out, him having developed a selective deafness.

. . .

There's been angry public response to those in public positions breaking their own rules. I need to catch up on walking routes for books and magazines. In case I get stopped, my publisher gives me a legal letter explaining I am working. Walking and writing now run the risk of a criminal record.

I go north to cover some routes for publication next year, to show the right season – there's no use showing Ingleborough in full winter garb when the article appears in June. I take Scout, initially for the day, but as restrictions relax and the country approaches something like normal, we have multi-day camps. He likes this, in the tent, snuggled in his own sleeping bag. We have some big days, reach the high points of several counties, saunter through dales and valleys, walk the borders of Scotland, England and Wales. The big hills adding muscle to Scout's drivetrain, crags expanding his balance and dexterity. He moves elegantly, thoughtfully studying the way ahead, choosing the right line. I like routes that are off the beaten path, the going hard work at times, scrambling up narrow clefts, navigating across featureless moors, the thighs and calves screaming, the heart hammering. I'm breathing a little heavier and the cough is still with me; my body's failing resilience struggling to fight it off. I'm certainly not as fit as I was a year ago at assessment. I develop a hill ascent process. Walk for a hundred metres then rest until my heart rate returns to something like normal and my breathing becomes restful, then I take a deep breath that pops my lungs and repeat the whole process. I invest in a shiny watch that tells me heart rate, breathing, sleep, goodness knows what else, plus it tracks my position and has an emergency call setting if I keel over. I become obsessed with heart rate, that red line that I crash into so easily. Scout has a new technique, romping ahead, then waiting until I catch up and my energy levels replenish. It's a good deal for him, each time he gets a treat.

A young man seeking release from the pandemonium of his world. We would not find him for he had chosen another wood, a different oak tree with a clear view of home. He got his release, the family holding it for the rest of their days.

Our search area was Wombwell Wood, an ancient forest mentioned in the Domesday Book. Dog walkers come at daybreak; some hurry away to desks, others drift between trees and conversations, their words left to litter the leafy floor. There are trees hanging from the sky, beech and hornbeam, chestnut and cherry. A glade of Scots pine and golden larch, the ground full of green and yellow curls. A thick, soft pile of rusting mast and golden leaf from autumn fall, for tiny feet to kick and crawl through. The edges fringed with hedge of hawthorn and berries of black and red. Primrose and dog rose and rising spires of purple foxglove and tomorrow's nettle soup, and today's cheese and bread. A crab apple for kids to eat and no doubt later bellyache instead of sleep. And oaks whose low branches float over cupules of acorns for little ones to keep, and bluebell drifts as far as the eye can see. At weekends, children sprout like mushrooms and by the hottest part of the day dens have been constructed, traps set and battlements made to repel the marauders. Mounds of crisp crumbly leaf are gathered for soft landings from black boughs, the loamy air filling with squeals and tears. Little girls totter in yellow beams like firefly in a golden sky.

Early afternoon, families drift on the warm air mingling with the speckled wood, orange tip and comma. Glades of sunlight are sought for tartan blankets, sandwiches passed, egg and cress; bottles of fizzy pop crack like dry twigs, and flasks of milky coffee decant into plastic cups. There's chatter and laughter. Above. The mottled sky. On thick black limbs that plunge out of vivid green and patches of powder blue, a sycamore seed, twirling through space until the sun draws long shadows and cool air to push people home and continue the happiness in manicured gardens.

As darkness gathers, youth steps away from the hands that still reach out, and quietly, slowly, make their way in shadows. Furtive glances reaching back, bottles and cans clinking in plastic bags, as the future merges into the trees and follows the track through to the old quarry. Picking tree fall along the way to make the fire then sit and play their songs, make love, pass the bottle and the twist and the needle into the long night.

Early afternoon, we move into the woodland quietly, opening ourselves to the resonance within. Scout stands gently by my side listening to the noises and looking at me; I guess he's asking why we are here. 'Find him out.' He begins the journey through his own world, moving like a shadow through the flicker of light and shade on the leafy ground, his bell adding to bird calls and drawing eyes as he passes unseen through the space, his free-wheeling movement graceful, present.

The wood is buzzing with life; families and friends dot the woodland floor, feasts set out, cool boxes with beer and ice cream. Scout veers close to these pockets of delights. Every so often he glances over to see if I am watching to see if he can get away with a sidle over to the picnic in hope of a morsel. It's going to be a long search, so I let him have these little moments then pull his mind back to the job.

Scout covers a lot of ground working our way to the quarry. I need to check there in case the missing person has fallen. There is the acrid tang of fire hanging in the air; I don't want Scout injured so I tell him to lie down in the dark coolness beneath a spreading oak. The quarry floor is covered with boulders; the fire still smoulders from last night's reveries, charred wood going from black to blue to grey. Bottles and cans litter the undergrowth, containers of junk food poke out from thorns and nettles. I'm scanning carefully until I spot what I guessed would be here. A silver line in the grass, a syringe. Once I have my eye in there are others, and twists of silver foil, used condoms, and wipes. I pick my way through people's good times, Scout shifting position under the tree to keep me in sight, keeping me safe. I do not want him in this place. There are human faeces and discarded clothing but it's days if not weeks old. Rusty oil drums, old barbed wire fencing, an old van; bramble and nettle consume it all. I can't see any disturbance but call Scout and run him around the top of the quarry to see if he picks anything up. There's nothing. We head back into the clean woodland, summer pouring into my brain pushing out the rancid play space.

We work for two hours, with a couple of short breaks to catch our breath. We take ten minutes' rest after two hours, refuel, check our coverage, messages, reset our minds. We'll keep this up until we find, or clear the area, or get stood down. If need be, we can stay out for twenty-four hours unsupported.

Clearing strips of the wood like a ploughman – turning at the edges and walking back – we move through the data fields of people's lives. We have one final stretch and we will be clear. The map shows a pond ahead of us, outside our search area, on our way back to control. If there is water, it will be a good place for Scout to have a cooling dip and unwind.

There are other areas to search, centred around the control van that sits in the place the missing person was last seen. The search managers have expanded the search out from this point, the police bringing more intelligence in, behavioural profiles adding further to the list of possible places, islands of trees, fields and small hamlets along thin sinewy roads.

Another forty minutes brings us close to the ponds; I know this, not because I can see them, but because Scout is beginning to range farther ahead, glancing back to see if I am going to check him, the smell of the water pulling him in. He breaks off to investigate a human scent. It's a plimsoll, child size. I pull him back to our trail with a pointed finger. Ahead I see the base of a line of trees on a long bank separating the wood from where the ponds should be.

We've cleared the area, so I radio in nothing found and tell them we are taking some time to decompress and get some food and drink. We aren't wanted as yet, so we'll take a gentle walk back to control. I don't mention the pond.

I can't see the water, but Scout is doing his little dance, running up to me, air barking, imploring me to release him for a swim. I'm wary of letting him go beyond my sight – the van in the quarry, all that barbed wire and needles. A little longer I tell him. He gets more manic, the forest canopy ringing with his barking, the forest floor gouged by his paws; golden leaf and loam spiral up through sunbeams. The bank is in view and the long stand of beech holding sentry along the top. I can't hold the line any longer so give him the permission to go. As soon as the letter G leaves me, he's gone. He doesn't go over the bank as I expected but veers off to the left disappearing like a shadow. Maybe a couple of seconds pass, but it's lost in what happens next.

It begins with silence. That, I will always remember. Then the splash. It must be a full belly flop dive into the water, cymbals crashing in the trees; the boughs, I fancy, sway back and forth as the sound wave pulses through. How high he had been when he launched I can only guess. I start for the gap only to be stopped by the next wave, a growling anger welling up from the other side of the bank. A wall of incrimination spreading out along the top, tumbling down to hold my feet in place. Real anger, people shouting, words rolling over the bank and spreading out about my feet. I can see the choppy green water, the edge of the pond, and a man standing waving his arm wildly, his mouth throwing globs of white spittle out, flecks spuming into the air falling on the broken surface of the pond. I can see a big black box behind him, the name 'Shakespeare' in blue, and a fishing rod. I can see Scout, his finest breaststroke. His body relaxed and cutting through the water, not a care in the world, looking around, perplexed at the noise. His eyes catch mine, eyebrows bobbing up and down. He changes course, swims away from me, his back legs pushing water behind him. There is a sign, proclaiming the first fishing match since the end of lockdown, asking people to keep a distance and have a wonderful time.

The shouting has not stopped. I pull back into the shadows and scramble up the bank, peering over the top. The ponds are lined with anglers, and all of them, all, are on their feet, heads bent forward, some punch the air like boxers in the ring, others frantically lift tackle clear of the water, reel in lines, pull keep nets, empty, on to dry land. Utter pandemonium. People are coming from elsewhere, some laughing, pointing at Scout still cleaving a way down the centre of the water without the slightest concern. A man tries to grab Scout, he gives him an easy swerve; another tries, almost falls in, older men pulling him back, the man blowing red cheeks.

I can't let this go on. If I call him from my side of the bank, they might grab him as he gets out. I have to go and get him. I'm in black, my team badge from a distance could be mistaken for a police badge, and if I wave my radio around, they might just assume, and that will dampen any vigilantes. Stepping through the gap I try to look as though I've just arrived. Scout is still swimming, people are still shouting, some are looking around to see who the blasted dog belongs to. Their eyes fall on me. I act all nonchalant, commanding Scout to swim around the perimeter of the pond. Anglers stare hard. I tell the nearest we are on a police search – technically true – and Scout needs to check the pond. A second angler steps away and a ripple of soft words flow around the pond; every angler clears the water of tackle and steps back from the edge. Silence falls. All eyes on Scout.

It's unlikely there is a body, but in case there is I guide Scout through the water. He glances left and right as he makes long graceful sweeps, occasionally chomping down on a bubble. Someone says the dog must be tasting the water. I continue the charade for a few more minutes then tell him to get out, pulling him on to the path, his body corkscrewing water across fishing tackle and blackening the path. 'Good lad.' I say this loud enough for all to hear.

I raise a hand and say thank you, then head for the gap, trying not to run, nodding to onlookers who follow us with wide eyes and open mouths. We reach the safety of the trees and away from the first fishing match since lockdown.

The trees are spaced further apart here, giving dappled clearings for Scout to weave in and out of. Feeling the blue sky above is like bathing in clean fresh air. Sunbeams and midges dance with the shadows, the light sifting the leafy reds and golds. Yellow leaf litters against the black of old trees. I close my eyes and take a deep breath, my mood lifting as nature pours its ages into my lungs. There is a gentle slope down to a small stream; at the top a tall beech watches over forest life, thick copse of oak and willow square off the sides; beyond is the horizon, clear above the canopy. I fancy the tree seems inviting, pleased I might choose it, let the search ease out of my bones and the anglers become a smile, take on some food, check the map for the way back, gain a few moments' rest. Scout scampers down to the stream, his paws rustling through dry leaf, the woodland's happiness filling the space, silver baubles lifting into the air to dance in the light as he enters the space.

The beech puts its arms around me, telling me to breathe slow and let the tension ease. As I get food out Scout comes powering up, his eyes fixed on his food flowing into his bowl, his nose in before I set it down. Finished, he lies at my feet to share what I have. A lump of cheese, some pie, some fruit. I share what I have with Scout, scolding him once again for never sharing his, ruffle his hair and release him to chase water beams.

A shadow moving to my left pulls. A young couple walking along a path high above the stream; heads come together every few beats, they kiss, walk on, kiss. Then turn and face each other. Two girls. They look so in love. One lifts a foot behind her, pulls the other close, closing the space, kisses, a long kiss that needs eyes closed and hands tight around soft clothes, a fingertip feels life on the precious skin and soft down of a neck. Heads press together, eyes lock. I think a smile. I smile. In the middle of this glorious wood, it's the most beautiful moment of the day; the trees sense it, the leaf flickers as a breeze whispers through. They walk on arm in arm, then around waists. I think that is how love should be.

Above I can hear birdsong. Different tunes for different birds I think; wish I knew more so I could tell who was wooing who. From the trees far behind, children scream and shout and laugh, the sheer joy of life, being young, not having to be someone. I get a brief passing of beech sap and cool water, feeling their way through the woodland. Thin branches tentatively dance, not sure if the music will continue, dazzling the floor. I absorb it all, become one with the day.

It is the road, slowly coming into view from years past. I try and clasp the meaning, moving through rooms in my mind. A friend's house. There, just after the bend, set back, the small garage at the side. She doesn't live there now. Now I have the meaning of it all.

The last time I had seen her she acted strangely, urgently moving to sit with me, putting her arm through mine, telling me how much she appreciated me as a friend, her normal closed-down reserve cast aside. She'd been through a lot of pain, every member of her family gone, relationships shattered after a few months, sometimes weeks. She found it hard to connect with people, was the most private person I knew, the walls of her life heavily guarded and fortified with few words or contact. I felt privileged to be counted as a friend; once appointed you weren't ever leaving. She had a flamboyant side that attracted beautiful women who lived on the periphery of her world, private women that had a vulnerability that fitted her need to be strong.

Three weeks after I saw her, she'd phoned, left a message for me to call. Two weeks after that I heard she'd hung herself, in the garage, the one I could see just after the bend in the road, set back, at the side of the house.

She'd taken control of the one thing she could, spending the final few days phoning friends to tell them how much they meant to her, choosing the ones to take in those final hours. She was saying thank you. I love you. Goodbye.

I hadn't returned her call. Hadn't given her that final gift of friendship. And there are times when I think about that and close my eyes. And there are times when I smile and think about the mountain days we had, the drenching rain, scouring winds and magical sunsets. And there are times when I get angry with her for leaving. And there are times when I don't think of her at all. And there are times when I cry.

It is painful for me to settle happenings like that. They remain constant companions. It's why I have a tough time with suicides; I see and know what the person leaves behind in those who remain. It isn't just memories. There is also guilt.

I take my time getting Scout comfortable in my van, give him a good brush, clean his jacket, pass him a few treats, then head over to control. There is plenty of daylight. Still, the inside of the van burns bright with lights and screens. Search managers watch ground sections moving on a map, take notes, listen to radio calls, chat with police. Some sections are back and, like us, waiting for the next deployment. I go through what we have covered, upload my track file. One of the dogs has moved on to a second area. I'm certain the missing person wasn't in our area when we searched. We're told to wait for another deployment. I can't decide whether to tell them about the fishing match. If I say nothing and they get a complaint it won't be good. I tell them they might get a complaint. Silence falls with a thud. The search manager puts his pen down, looks up; everyone does.

'What about?'

'Well, Scout interrupted some people, they might complain.' I'm wanting to keep this as brief as possible, knowing where this could go.

'How do you mean, interrupted?' The final word is underlined, in italics, in bold. People can smell blood and begin to wander over.

'He jumped into a pond at the end of the search. To cool off.' I add the last bit in the hope that ends the conversation. It doesn't.

'Why would that upset people?' These are old hands at the game and can smell a major screw-up from a long, long way off. Masters in the psychology of humiliation, they know when a team member is trying to cover up some misdemeanour. A golden opportunity. Legends are built on such.

'Well, nothing really. They were doing something. Taking part in something. Scout sort of disturbed something. A little. A bit.'

'Doing something. Taking part in something. Sort of disturbed something. That's a lot of somethings.'

People are now several layers deep behind me. I'm trapped and I've run out of excuses. I spill the beans and tell them about Scout swimming in the fishing match. A wide smile spreads across the search manager's face. He looks around at everyone, his eyes sparkling.

'Gritstone.'

Autumn approaches and the pandemic recedes. People pour outdoors, tents litter the landscape, vans block field gates and any scrap of land that can take wheels. Businesses are still closed, giving waiting hands lots of free time. The definition of staying local is stretched, transgressions fill the newspapers, national parks maintain their exclusivity, the golf courses let walkers stroll. The hills are alive.

Van life and wild camping are growth hobbies. Driven by social media influencers enticing people with a get-away-from-it-all confection of self-sufficiency and adventure. For those that can afford it, it's a cottage in the Cotswolds, or Cornwall, or a 'remote and idyllic' Welsh valley with no power, artisan bakes, chair making and village life. For many, it's converting a van on the drive, or a tent as big as a bungalow, and all the goodies to go with it. For some, erecting a tent in the dark will be the least of their worries.

The toll on teams begins to build inexorably. Mountains are overrun with campers, makeshift camps litter lake shores like autumn leaves, abandoned at the first drop of rain. Tents, chairs, food, beer, all left where they were dropped; trees denuded of branches; fires left to smoulder; barbecues send fires sweeping across moors. It's clear these are people who have only a tenuous connection to the outdoors. Social media sites are awash with clips of the togetherness of a fireside camp, orange flames burning glowing faces backed by the darkness of the night. Old-timers push *leave no trace*, landowners despair, keyboard warriors rant.

The romance of being away from urban life is hard to resist. Teams are still working with reduced numbers, and the grinding away of physical health is beginning to show. Many have coughs, the fear of Covid raising its head every time they clear their lungs. Still, we all take tests, wear the masks and goggles and gloves, our bodies sealed inside sweat-inducing man-made fibres. It isn't pleasant. Chest infections, the wheezing, the feeling lungs and heart will explode, lugging a stretcher and casualty across rugged terrain in all weathers. There is no one else. So, we carry on.

I take my annual fitness test. Cut Gate in seventy-five minutes, well within the time, a nice amble for myself and Scout. A week later I push myself up Parkin Clough. It hurts; my heart thumps away like an old steam pump, my lungs struggle to keep up a constant delivery of oxygen. I stop twice to get my breath, hand outstretched against a tree, upper body bent over, counting out the seconds till my breathing calms. Scout, well above me, stands watching, his look intense. Finally, I make it to the trig pillar, a finger pressing the stopwatch. Twenty-nine minutes and thirty-eight seconds.

I've had the same cough since early summer and don't seem to be able to shift it; I get a few days clear and then it's back. I'm going through bottles of cough mixture with no lasting effect. I'm beginning to suspect I might have asthma. With the depleted numbers the team doesn't need to be another man down, so I buy more cough syrup, carry on huffing my way up hills and say nothing.

A second lockdown arrives. This one is promised to be shorter so kids can see granny at Christmas, from the government that encouraged people to eat out, now seen by many as fuelling the rise in infections and deaths. With winter approaching and the traditional flu season about to begin, experts believe there is a real danger of the hospitals being overwhelmed. But experts are not in vogue this year, their message spoiling many a party. Team members who work in the NHS relay horror stories of what is happening inside the hospitals. No one stands on the doorstep clapping.

I head south with Scout, driving through the national park. Coming the other way the roads are full of builders' vans driving into the city; everyone is remodelling. Driving so far from home is stressful, even with a pass. I chat to Scout about the route we will walk. The walk takes us across the face of a limestone cliff, named the most dangerous walk in Britain on social media. I wouldn't go that far, but for some it will be testing. I'm interested to see what Scout will make of it – he's good on crags, has no fear of ledges and knows not to go over the edge of a cliff. Here, the exposure is total, the path a few feet wide. There is a dense cloud inversion in the valley below; the photos are incredibly atmospheric, perfect for the magazine. We are literally walking on the clouds. Scout trots happily along, his mountain legs in control, more interested in scent than the crown of trees we walk over.

The landscape is deserted, the heritage centre is locked and empty; the day has an apocalyptic feel. Farms have re-routed public paths away from barns and housing, signs directing to a new alternative. Some paths are completely blocked, gates locked, slurry spread knee deep in front of stiles; access points are rotting, the fabric of the countryside disintegrating.

We rest with a view of the cliff we traversed early in the day. The bench is by an amusement park, everything closed up; gondolas swing high above suspended in time. I feel like we're the last beings on earth. The air is still crystal clear. No planes fly, no traffic noise pushes through the silence, only the birds sing. Scout is in the moment, eyes closed, chin on paws, completely relaxed. I'm beginning to learn about living in the moment from him.

Christmas sees lockdown lifted.

The local handlers take the opportunity for some training in Grindsbrook. There is deep snow and blue skies, clouds that hug the tops of the crags and a bitter wind. People are out in droves, asking numerous questions about walks across the Kinder Scout plateau. Few have a map; the number of times someone waves a smartphone is legion; they jab it with their finger to wake it from its cold slumber, point at the red line across the green pastel landscape they've downloaded on a free app. A small icon blinks their position. If we ask if they have a torch, they wiggle the phone in front of us, smiling. Technology the answer to all hills. What would we know. Few are clothed to last more than an hour on the top if things go wrong. It could be a busy day.

A handler scribes out an area with a finger. The path in the bottom of the valley, the gullies east and west, the sky above. Black, white and blue. I want to work Scout for a good period of time, it isn't often we get these conditions. There's a good wind running up the valley, so we zigzag our way up through the area. I manage our time with regular stops. It's hard work for me, post-holing through deep drifts, even harder for Scout when he keeps disappearing underneath the blanket of snow. I conveyor feed him pemmican to keep his energy levels up, the block of fats and carbs swallowed with gusto. He's very comfortable and enjoying the conditions. I keep high, forming the top boundary of each zigzag so he can swing down the steep slope then work back. When we hit a scoured section of moor, the tips of frozen heather forming a hard skin, we move more easily and push on. The valley floor has groups of denim-clad visitors trying not to get muddy. We have untarnished snow, a firm wind, blue skies and clouds I could almost touch. And silence. Only when we move is there the sound of my boots creaking through snow.

The drifts give our muscles a good workout. Scout has stopped growing upward now and is filling out, his chest broad, limbs powerful. He doesn't ask for help if he falls into a hole, just looks at me and pulls himself out. There's a rock outcrop in the centre of the area that he snaps his nose to, then slaloms down and vanishes behind. Then he's back, scanning the landscape, checking where I am, giving his double take when he finds me, plans a route to me to tell me he's found. When I get there, he's waiting. The dogsbody is still. The ball appears and Scout, the body and the ball get engulfed in an avalanche of white powder. Snow splays out as Scout lands, his paws sinking deep. It's a beautiful day.

By the end of the year, we've worked another 600 hours, Scout has attended twenty-one call-outs and found people in distress. It's been a year of finding our feet. We've done well. My health has taken a battering, as have many others. We aren't fatigued yet, but how long teams of volunteers can keep working under these conditions is becoming a question.

2021

The first day of lockdown, the first call-out of the year. A young person, vulnerable and missing. We search an old quarry that night, burnt-out cars, metal and glass everywhere. Scout cuts a paw, though I don't know this until we have stood down. He comes over and holds it up for me; he'd carried on until the end. We make another donation to the local vet's luxury Tuscan villa fund and take a month off to put our paws and feet up.

Six days into the year Covid is rampant again and the country has entered its third national lockdown.

I work on writing, putting the next book to bed – *1001 Walking Tips* is part of a series covering outdoor activities. I've never been a fan of jargon, or the wannabe, we've seen too many of them recently. There's a lot of online criticism of people who've made mistakes, got rescued, wore the wrong clothing; it's something I am very much against. The book is full of simple tips – my experience, knowledge, mistakes I've made; it aims to get people out walking safely to have an enjoyable day. Walking and learning how to care for and respect our environment, and each other, should be part of the school curriculum, but we seem trapped by an education system that mines students as products.

The lockdowns have shown me the beauty of our local environment, of taking time to observe, of slowing down. We are studying how we as a family can change the way we live, even escaping north to smaller communities with more space, local shops and services. The geographical side of this fades; moving won't change things, we have to begin by changing ourselves.

It is the beginning of a search for a life that has a different focus. A great deal of this stems from Alison, who isn't afraid of exploring spiritual answers to the questions she has. It's led her to Buddhism, yoga and meditation, and fifty years as a vegetarian. I see the evidence, her values in her approach to the world. A calmness underpins her life – she experiences the light of the day and rarely is drawn into the shadows.

I get a knock on the door. Out of my study window I see the team Land Rover driving off, curtains twitching up and down the street. There's a square parcel wrapped in newspaper on the step. It's heavy. Unwrapped, it's a block of gritstone painted gold, as are now my hands.

The team has its AGM that evening, online. The main event, the awards for the best screw-ups. Scout's swim through the fishing match gets rewarded with the top prize, the Golden Gritstone. It's a great honour, one to be proud of, and added to the Golden Turd award from the dogs for the iPhone debacle on Gray Crag.

Now that all the restrictions have lifted, we set to preparing for our upgrade assessment in November. With Steve, we work on refining direction control, getting Scout to cover more ground and access out-of-the-way places without me having to take him. At the assessment we need to show that we have progressed. As we work through the search area, I remain at a vantage point to move Scout around me; it's less walking and a greater number of rests save energy. I still cannot shake the cough, and now I have a tight chest. The cold does not make things easier.

The dying days of winter see the season throw one last hurrah.

… and walk down to the bridge, the soft water taking the valley one grain at a time. The snowstorm has abated. Now we are in a winter wonderland of blue sky, the valley thick with virgin snow, untainted. Everything sparkles in the sunlight. The wind races through the confines of the narrow valley cutting through the glassy air. Massive lumps of sugar litter the landscape; blue shadows form in their lee. The further down we go, the further back in time, the higher the crags above reach to the sky.

I take a moment to settle myself, keeping the lead free of my tension. My lungs scrunch up with the cold, triggering a dry coughing fit that rasps tissue. Scout searches my face. In his deep brown eyes, the clouds flit by; the more I look the more I seem to peer into a galaxy without end. Calm myself, lose the tension and the fear. Search the area and do not; do not look for a body. Work the plan. The chest eases, the mind stops thrumming. Scout looks into the valley, his nose twitching as he collects scent. He turns, puts a paw on my foot and looks at me. We're ready.

Closing my eyes, I see both of us moving through the pristine space. A dozen faces crowd my mind, pulling and pushing, laughing, turning away. Old words hold me in a place I did not want to be. I should have stood up for myself more, should have turned my back. The lost years lay heavy in my stomach, my eyes screw tighter. All those years ago and still I hold on. Another cough, dry, rattling bones.

A sharp sting on my cheek brings me back; I feel the wetness with my finger. Scout is peppered with countless sparkling stars locking my vision and mind, willing them not to melt away. The valley is banded white, black and blue. Scout looks at me.

'Find him out.' He is gone, absorbed into black and white.

The wind bullies as I step in its path, putting its shoulder to me, throwing my balance as I pick a way across boulders trying to keep Scout in sight. All my mental and physical energy is converted into staying upright. I dance in short bursts from one slippery podium to the next, then rebalance, the chest heaving, my back wrapped in steel rods. If I don't break a leg it will be a miracle. I watch Scout as he gracefully taps a path across the sugary dance floor, cutting across the wind as it barrels through us. Sometimes he takes a high vantage point, looking majestic and commanding, his nose sampling particles as they stream towards that pink tongue pointing into the wind, nostrils flaring, eyes half closed, luxuriating in scent. His head tilts sideways as the data flows through his chambers; he ponders, sifts and works the data with his algorithm. Analysis over, he moves on. Occasionally he looks back at me, something that is becoming more common, for what reason I'm unsure.

We drink from the brook; he snorts, I brain freeze. Take some energy, pemmican, his head twisting for more before he's even swallowed, eyes darting from mine to treat pocket and back, a thick band of drool sinking a well into the snow. Teasing him, I can feel him trying to attract my attention, then see his nose on the edge of my vision. Me, the bag carrier, flicks a piece in the air. Scout's eyes following the trajectory, the morsel vanishing into his open mouth.

We work quietly into the labyrinth of scent. I direct with whistles, arms outstretched, progress choreographed effortlessly. There are times we slow, his attention drawn to scent on the ground, on a rock, in its shadow. A look calls me; I'm already on my way. '*Look*', he's saying. The snow is pristine, the intricate matrix of interlocking flakes easily visible, though no physical human signs. Scout knows there is human scent here; I know he knows. There are pulses of wind, ice crystals blowing over the surface, moving scent around in iridescent bands. Shadows move across, the cloud blocking sun momentarily plunging us into ice. I feel skin cells detaching from flesh. The snow has pushed up the valley, white caps break waves, shadow adding another dimension for scent to collect. Ahead lies the high wall of rock calving off Stable Stones Brow. Between us a land of bumps and hollows, outcrops of rock and scraggly vegetation. Scout has turned his attention to the wall and has been pecking the wind. He has something. We must be at the extreme boundary of the scent cone. I slow down, lighten the voice, soften the words. Let him know – work close and work the cone.

There are fervid stops, the nose probing the invisible human presence, the head lifting into the air, sharp violent snorts, eyes in rapture, the detritus of human flesh sifted. At times he will move on, then return, draw in more scent, the brain processing molecules, the algorithm choosing – yes, tell, or go.

If it is a yes, his movements are deliberate, his whole being held in the embrace of those invisible boundaries. I give him time, allow his body to settle, his mind quieten, until, like a key in a lock he sloughs off the waiting human world and steps across the threshold into his own domain. It is breathtaking and beautiful to watch, offering his soul to be absorbed by the space. Tentatively at first, testing for permission and acceptance, listening to the cacophony of smells, slowly inching along the human spoor. I gaze spellbound by the unfolding grace.

'Find him out.'

He checks me, I repeat, smiling, pointing to the ground hoping he will get a lock on the breadcrumb of scent. Scout snorts, begins snuffling around the scent dump; I'm sure that's what we have, and with no footprints the source is elsewhere. He moves from one binary boundary to the other. There must be a minute number of cells here; hard to put them together as the same collection, but he's sure. Slowly, whatever is beyond begins to pull Scout away from me. I stay downwind, find a large flat boulder to scan the waves of snow he begins to surf. Winter's last hurrah.

'Find him out.'

Scout moves methodically over the outcrops, choosing his paw place-ments with care, drawing a safe passage for both of us. He hovers here and there to check the strength of the scent, vibrating his tongue on the surface that has drawn his loving attention. Then adjusts course, right or left, always in the scent cone, always moving forwards. No matter the distance he will deliver me to the source.

Across rock, in and out of dips, he plots a line to the wall. At last, he stands at the foot and begins probing the base, sometimes returning to make further analysis of what his nose has seen there, then moves on. Left and right boundaries much closer together now, his step more definite as the scent grows stronger, the cone narrower. A step or two back from the wall, nose in the air, eyes searching for a line up. He's seen the ledges, and a line, so begins his pitch up the natural staircase, his paws gripping rough stone, whisps of snow floating metres above my head, twisting and spiralling on the breeze. His muscles twitch and tense as he works and tests holds. Sometimes he reaches too far, and my muscles tighten; I have to work hard not to shout. At a fissure he sticks his nose deep into the blackness, snowflakes dazzling the air around his head, rainbows dancing like stardust. I can see a cloud of evaporation lifting out of the crack; he leans back, looks, sniffs inside, sniffs outside, then looks above. There's a rising rake running up to an edge; he begins to work a way up, sometimes pulling sometimes pushing, moving easily. He's high now. The edge comes into clear focus in my mind map.

I'm silent, fingers stabbing the air, breathing held for too long. At the top he lifts himself over with his front paws, the back legs scratching at the surface till they find purchase, haunches bulging with strength. The whole of the valley has shrunk across a wide void I dare not transgress.

Silently, I pray. *Please don't fall, please don't fall.*

With one great heave, clumps of snow clouding the air, he tips over the top and is gone, the only sign of his presence the gouged snow and bared rock and a falconer's bell tinkling in the sky. He is unharmed. He is still searching.

Dancing across boulders, I want to yelp with pride. Something to my right moves, a shadow scudding low across the snow, the light sucked into the darkness, wind screams, a blizzard swirls around me pressing my body into grey snow. The world shifts into monochrome. I can still hear his bell moving into the wind, then it's silenced by a deep rumble from roiling clouds. I'm off balance and crouching, fingertips plunging through snow feeling for solid rock, feet shuffling for a flattish surface; the cold burns my hands and bones. Darkness falls, the air hanging in heavy stillness. I pray for Scout.

Silence.

The squall passes and the sky lifts. Great shards of light push away the cold shadows, brightening the air bouncing blue from the snow. Scout's presence has gone, his pawprints wiped clean with fresh snow. In the distance sleigh bells get nearer and louder until he is there at the edge of the ledge. Maybe it's the wind and the snow, but my face is wet and beaming with love for this little man. Steam plumes around me, lungs finally free to breathe. He scans the snow field. Sweeping south he spots me, a look of surprise crossing his face, then he measures the distance and plots his route and begins his descent, concentrated and purposeful, picking footholds, shifting weight to maintain balance. At a large boulder he stops, checks our relative positions, recalibrates, moves on, head first. I move towards him, saving him energy. A Scout-length from me he lifts his head and emits a single loud bark. I can see right down his throat, the corrugations of bone, pink and black flesh, the long tongue safe in its lair. His indication ricochets off the crag; he's already heading back, a tangle of snow the only sign he was at my feet. I follow, his indication still ringing the rocks behind me. I pick my way through rock and drift, some post-holing, a lost leg now and again – I'm trying my best to follow his path, but he's better at this than me. At times, my mass and pace accelerate me frighteningly close to crashing into the ground. I survive, finally reaching the base of the rock long after he has passed beyond. I can still hear his bell.

Snowpack tumbles around me. Scout is back, peering over the edge, watching me with those hooded eyes. He says nothing. There's a ramp to the right, probably a sled-way that leads up to whatever it is he's standing on. More pristine snow to be post-holed, working my groins, my lungs burning. Scout barks his frustration.

'Just wait.'

He nips my hand to speed me up, gives me the once over, satisfying himself I'm still capable, then he's off along the wide ledge, his prints obliterating the ones he made earlier. I can see his post holes in the deeper snow, and the groove his chest made.

'Find him out.'

A token command just to say I am here. He doesn't stop but gives a bark of admonition, his tail swishing madly – he is so up for this, as happy as I have ever seen him. Another bark. His tail vanishes.

Silence.

Angels pass. Bell chimes sprinkle the ether. His face comes into view; the black, white and tan are clear against the snow-spattered rock, snow on his snout. He peers surreptitiously round the corner of the boulder, just his head, looking at me. Then a bark, bringing snow sliding off the rock, engulfing his head. I laugh. He smiles. Shakes the snow off, moves a pace forward, barks, thumps the snow. He's really angry. I half walk, half run, behind the rock. He's sat, tail brushing snow aside, his head held high and proud. His eyes pull mine down to a gap between the rocks, the surface stamped with paw prints.

'Show me.'

He pulls my eyes to the gap, releases a silent bark. A bivvy bag.

'You clever boy!' His toy launches into the sky. He corkscrews up – mouth open, eyes wide, suspended for a second in the blue – then drops, the snow strafing a circle around us, the toy safe.

My words ring across the valley. The body rises from his hibernation, shaking off snow and rubbing life back into limbs. He was the anomaly in the landscape, the very tip of the cone. The warmth from his body and the bright sun had lifted his scent to catch the thermals and wind, carrying it out into the valley. The colder air then drew it down the gritstone crag and over the boulder field – dropping scent caches as it went, catching on rock and plant, settling, drifting with blasts of cold air – finally reaching the scent dump where Scout first found it and followed its binary code to the source. It is a super find, hard work and technically demanding.

It's been a long haul, my limbs are tired, my breathing needs a rest. I sit, taking in all the points Scout found scent, working out how the scent had moved, shifted through all the levels of the snowy land. The boulders around me, at the base of the crag, remind me of my fall, lying in the snow wondering if I had just dreamed of a dog coming to me, knowing, somehow, all would be well. The thought catches me. Everything that happened today is a thread that stretches across all those years when I stepped across that small brook running through the snow into the darkness. And beyond that.

Scout drops his toy on my foot with a thud. I'd forgotten about him, being wrapped in the past. I pitch the toy high. For a moment he watches, waiting until it reaches its nadir where it hangs for a beat for Scout to launch himself – the hind legs springing him upwards, mouth opening, eyes locked, the descent into the thick snow. He tosses the ball to me, crouches low, eyes tracking the ball as I wave it slowly, his object of desire. Nothing comes close for him. The ball twirls in the air, its rope twisting in my fingers, then slingshots into the snow, his nose driving the ridges of a furrow, sunlight bouncing off the crystals flickering reds, blues, yellows and greens. Triumphant he lifts his prize, rolls on his back and lifts the trophy high above him in adoration.

. . .

The days have warmed. Spring is vibrant and green. We are in the North for a few days completing work on some multi-day walks. It's quieter than I expected; most people are going abroad now the planes are back in the air, people trying their best to restart a normal life. Costs are rocketing; a pub charges me £9 for three sausages for Scout who makes them disappear in seconds before I've even put the ketchup on my home-made £22.50 burger. We don't call again.

We spend days exploring routes and views, the weather dry and warm, the landscape lively after the hard winter. Ever on duty, Scout calls me over to a shake hole as we ascend Ingleborough. I'd waved to the two cavers as they walked by during one of our breaks, and wondered how Scout would react to their scent. I'd kept an eye on them until they sank into the limestone underworld. Sure enough, he snaps to a shake hole, sniffs around and comes back to tell me he's found something but no body, running ahead pulling me along with his eyes. I feel the cold air rising from the hole – I can't smell them but fancy I can hear voices; Scout has the cavers. We spend a wonderful three days on the highest peaks, barren moors and the longest drystone walls I've ever seen. Descending back to camp in glorious golden sunsets.

Mid-summer I see the doctor. I am lucky: a newly qualified GP. She plays by the book, tests my chest, asks a few questions – how long, always dry, history, that kind of thing. She sends me for an X-ray that comes back clear, but she isn't happy. She can hear strange noises in my chest, rice crispies crackling. She asks more questions, speaks of red flags, refers me to the respiratory clinic. I don't expect to be seen quickly.

A few days after my referral I have an appointment. Mountain rescue has a long arm in the health service; many nurses, doctors and consultants are embedded in both. Perhaps I have a guardian angel, or maybe my number came up. I begin a series of examinations – breathing tests, timed walking, CT scans – then a list of possible causes is drawn up. Asthma scores high (all those stretcher carries wearing a mask), heart problems, biological infection (stretcher carries again), some type of fungus (stretcher carries), fibrosis. I become a regular at the hospital, my green Scarpa Mojitos resting on familiar lino in a variety of waiting rooms.

We continue honing strategy, big searches on the tough ground around the Chew Valley. Thursdays we stay close to home, work on detail, finesse.

It's easier on Scout than at Chew, shorter too so he gets lots of exciting finds. It's easier for me as well. My chest still has not cleared. We've refined the new way of working, shoving Scout further on to clear larger areas of land, allowing me to hold at vantage points; as Steve says, 'Why have a dog and do all the searching yourself?' I move a few hundred metres at a time, rest, get my breath back, slow the heart. Along the flat, traversing a hillside or crag, coming off the tops, I don't have a problem.

It isn't all grind, there is lightness. We stick a body down a fairy hole to see what Scout does. He catches the scent and drops down to the entrance. I can see him working through his library of scenarios until he gets to the day on Ingleborough, and he launches himself into the underworld.

After finishing an exercise Scout trundles ahead, freewheeling along the top of a crag only to return with an indication. He takes me 300 metres then drops off the edge. I find him sat watching two old boys having their lunchtime sandwiches by an old quarry hut, Bramley's Cot. They return his penetrating gaze, shuffling feet as his stream of saliva saturates the ground. Scout can't understand why they aren't sharing, cheese and pickle on Warburtons white. I call him away; the old boys keep eating, a hand on their sandwich box. Another time I send him on while I huff and puff my way to the top. We've the moor below Ashway Rocks to search, the wind coming up from the valley floor, rising over the top, leaving a dead space by the edge and dumping scent on the moor beyond the edge path. When I get to the top, he's coming back indicating a find. Another dance, so no body. It will be a scent dump I figure. He takes me to Ashway Stone, and a large pink dildo. I'm guessing there is definitely human scent. I leave it where it is. Coming back at the end of the exercise Scout rushes ahead. No one has claimed it, so Scout does, proudly carrying it in his mouth back to the Office.

We hire a cottage in summer, on Scotland's west coast. It's quiet, nestled in a small cove with mountains all around. Stalkers' paths take us through heather, dolphins come into the bay, convoys of VW transporters and RVs hunt in packs along the North Coast 500. We walk and swim, collect Lewisian gneiss. I try my hand at drawing and painting. Scout spends his days in the sea; we swim together, gliding through the smooth warm water, smiles on our faces, glances frequently exchanged.

Back home, I go on a health and fitness drive in preparation for assessment. Walking, running, dieting. Scout acts as pacemaker in the forest. Running is mind numbing. My head isn't in it, nor are my legs; I grind away the kilometres. We put in some long walks to improve our stamina, taking the train out then walking back home along the gritstone edges, moors and valleys. It's a good thirty kilometres so we begin with a full English at the station, Scout with a sausage butty, plus anything he cons out of me and anyone else, then we work our way up a beautiful ravine on to the moors. We cross the valleys, some rough terrain and some land where we can get speed. Scout ambles in front exploring scent in heather and between rocks. It's a beautiful day: the pink heather swarms across the moor; warm gritstone gives islands to sit back and enjoy the display of grey, green, pink, blue. White clouds drift idly across the sky. We saunter along the edges; it's midweek so quiet, a few climbers around, a few oldies stop for a chat. I've got Vibram FiveFingers on my feet, helping to reduce weight on my legs – they make a good talking point. Scout hugs the lip of the crag; I move easily, feel good, the landscape holding me softly.

Scout indicates, drawing me over to the very tip of Stanage Edge. He knows we're not working so I'm interested to see what he's found, probably a plastic bottle or a discarded glove. Once it was a lens cap dropped minutes before on Ronksley Moor. Today there is nothing. I stand looking out at the space that holds the valley; perhaps someone's scent has lifted over the top of the crag. All I can see are splatters of pink heather, green bracken, silver rock underneath a blue sky dappled with balls of cotton. I ask him to show me; he points to the gritstone. 'There's nothing here,' I say. I get the look as he sticks his nose down a wide crack. In the depths is a human head halfway down the chimney; I can't see a rope. I ask if they are okay. 'Stuck,' says the head. I tell him I'll call mountain rescue and begin sorting a grid reference while I give Scout his reward. My concern is the climber might slip out of the squeeze and plunge to the ground. I'm about to phone when the climber's friend appears, throwing into the crack a high-tech jacket which the climber uses to smear their way out of the jam. Ego restored.

The missing, lost and broken are the bread and butter of our work. The vulnerable are still finding life hard, and the police finding it just as hard to resource searches. Social media spreads word of missing individuals giving rise to groups undertaking searches and appealing for word of any possible sightings. It's understandable and well-meaning, though large numbers of untrained, unmanaged and ill-equipped people can cause problems –

important clues missed, scent obliterated. We try to stay clear but often the control sites are known, and at times we find ourselves on display.

A despondent person is missing, their vehicle located at a local beauty spot – moors, woodland and water making up the landscape. It becomes the control rendezvous for a multi-agency search: fire brigade, police, helicopters. Mountain rescue has multiple teams working in remote and difficult areas. Over a hundred members of the public are here, drawn by social media, some to offer help, others just to be here. They congregate on the approach to the control vehicles, discussing where the search should look, debating the movements of a person they know little of. The dogs search Win Hill from the summit trig, down wooded slopes, dropping to Ladybower Reservoir. We search for several hours, clearing areas. Late afternoon we are stood down. The missing person found out of our area. Deceased.

It becomes known that relatives are present in the crowd. They're gently moved away, police and team members keeping onlookers at bay. It's decided to extract the casualty to another location away from the crowd.

I take a slow walk back with Scout. People are lined each side of the access road, some milling around in the centre, lots of rucksacks, camouflage gear, phones taking photos. They begin to clap as Scout and I move through, the centre parting. This is not what I want. I just want to debrief and go home.

A man steps forward and puts his hand out to shake mine, his other hand grasping the woman's by his side. They look broken. I shake his hand because I can't think of anything else to do and try to move on. He says thank you, gently, his eyes apologetic, pleading. I look him straight on, and nod acknowledgement, recognising their presence and their loss, surmising this must be the relatives. He looks bewildered, in a world he could never have imagined, engulfed by pain. I walk on; the controller gathers me in and says that's the relatives. The encounter imprints deeply in my psyche.

The hospital keeps searching. It's difficult because I'm very much an outlier in terms of fitness. Normally patients they see have been stuck on a settee for a few years watching daytime television, their level of fitness well below someone who spends most of their time yomping across moors. I'm the anomaly.

I push myself in training and call-outs, saying nothing to anyone, but my mind is beginning to skip bits of information. I don't realise this until much later – likening it to turning two pages of a book instead of one, the narrative still continuing but not quite joining up. Worse, the black dog of depression is roaming through the house looking for me.

Scout's mind and body have reached their peak of performance, as I feel mine have begun to ebb away. It takes me longer now to get up the hill, more time and thought to cross the boulder field, more care needed at night. He stands looking across the landscape at my progress; he's stopped hurrying me, waits patiently for my arrival, insists on rest. We share water and treats. His confidence complete, he pays more attention to me these days, sure of the ground he stands on. At first, I thought he was annoyed with my slow progress, a human body no match for a mountain rescue Border collie. As time unfolded, I realised he sensed in me that which I had not. It wasn't impatience, it was care. He needed to be sure I was safe, that I was there in body and mind. He was watching over me. He knew.

Our upgrade will be in late autumn, in Wales. I'm not confident for three days on the hill, but I want this for Scout, he deserves to be amongst the best. I keep my head down and mouth closed, keeping the scent of failure from drifting off me. To boost confidence on the big Welsh hills I test my fitness. My ascent of Parkin Clough is hell. Even before I have left the road I'm struggling, my lungs screaming to stop, taking numerous pauses to get air into my lungs and cease the hammering in my chest. When I finally hit the summit, I press the stopwatch. Forty-nine minutes. The cut-off is thirty minutes; ten months ago, I took twenty-nine minutes. My confidence avalanches as I rest against the pillar trying not to make eye contact with people staring at me. Scout stands close by, searching my face. I say nothing to anyone.

The week of assessment is hectic; Friday will be our first day on the hill. I pack and repack, make lists, go over strategy with Steve and try to sleep.

Thursday morning I'm at the hospital for an update on all the tests, and, I'm hoping, some help with my breathing. My consultant and a team of specialists discussed my case that morning; all agree. The heart is fine. There is no sign of asthma or infection. I have asbestosis.

It isn't really a surprise, though I have held the thought at arm's length for many years. All those years in the steelworks, hacking away asbestos, making asbestos joints. The consultant tells me my lungs have the fibres and irreversible scarring has occurred and will keep occurring. It's taken almost half a century from my first day in the steel mill – the job for life – for it to get me. There is no cure, no stopping its onward progress. How long I have they cannot say, they don't know yet how fast it is spreading.

I drive down to Wales that evening. I remember nothing of the journey.

We get RAC Technical first. We find the bodies in good time, but my sense of position is off, at one point traversing the crag face while a clear path runs ten metres below. The second hill I struggle getting up. Like on the first hill I employ the strategy of ascent then rest while I work Scout around. We find all the bodies and again are in time, but my breathing is bad, and my heart is blowing for all it's worth. The assessors say I'm taking too long and need to be much smoother, moving through the area with energy. That night I look at my heart rate stats. The whole day has been spent way above my maximum heart rate; it's clear I cannot continue. Next morning, I walk away from the assessment. I feel terrible. I've let Scout down badly; now he will never be up there with the others, and he deserved to be. I say my thanks to everyone, struggling to keep the upset out of my words. On the drive back I pull into a forest clearing and walk into the trees with Scout. We find a fallen tree to sit on; I just stare ahead into the darkness, seeing only the pain of failure. The tears pour out.

Back home I tell Alison about the asbestosis. Nothing fits into the plans we had for the future, and what the time ahead holds is beyond our comprehension. We spend Christmas in a fog, neither knowing the what or when of it all.

With friends, I share what is happening. About the assessment, about the sense of failure, about ending it all, my hand on a switch putting me on a trajectory I have no control of. I don't want Alison to suffer caring for me, she doesn't deserve that.

Everything piles into the dark hole, a cauldron of resentments, anger, bullying and weakness that spirals me down to my darkest moment. I make plans, dig out an old climbing rope, write in my journal each day that suicide is the best option. But how without traumatising Alison?

A friend says the one thing I don't seem upset about is the asbestosis, the thing that has been done to me, and is killing me. She says, 'Don't you think that's odd? I'd be mad as hell.' After several decades of building a life without drink one day at a time, I'm planning my own death. All my experience, all my knowledge, is this really where I am? She was the partner of the girl I thought of just after Scout joined in the fishing match. She isn't gentle, tells me to get help, see the doctor, get some medication. She takes my hand off the switch.

I try to understand what is happening, diving into books on well-being as it's now called. I read about people having battles with their own demons. I listen to podcasts, collecting anything that will help me get from underneath the crushing weight. Bizarrely, I keep training with Scout, say nothing of this to anyone, other than Scout, who demonstrates things don't matter, past or present – all there is, is the now, this moment. I wish it was that simple I tell him. It is, he says.

We get called out one night for a missing vulnerable person with a history of suicide attempts. We search woodland and crags, other dogs searching high moors. We see areas rarely entered by the public, wonderful secret worlds of fantasy and magic. As dawn lifts, we stand down for day sections to continue. The missing person found later that day, having not survived the night.

I learn of a dog handler who has taken their own life, one of the people who assessed us when we became operational. I remember they always had a word of encouragement, a nudge in the right direction, and they were a loner. After learning of their death, I think about them a lot, how together they seemed, how no one knew. The Third Man who began training with Scout and I all those years ago has also gone. Taking their exits, leaving memories and a hole for those left behind.

With my doctor I talk through what is happening, being ruthlessly honest. She says there is lots of trauma in the emergency services from the last few years and mountain rescue would be no different. Plus, I've been told I'm dying from something that happened half a century ago. Have I factored that in? While she is gentle and understanding, she is brutally firm. I get some happy pills, and there is talking therapy. I'm unsure about talking to a stranger about what I see are my weaknesses. Each week the doctor calls and asks if I want to take my own life. Some weeks I say, sometimes. She ups the pills.

The therapy will take time to begin as resources are scarce. Covid and cutbacks all rolling into the perfect storm for mental health services. I'm unconcerned, the drugs seem to be having an effect; talking to a stranger about the stuff in my head, anger, resentments, petty squabbles with people who are not present in the room, is the last thing I want. To confront this would be to confront myself, and I'm increasingly unsure who the real me is.

That apologetic 'thank you', spoken softly, keeps running around my head; the look of desolation in those eyes makes me think of Alison, left alone, trying to work out what she could have done to prevent my suicide. And what about Scout, why does he deserve being abandoned?

Scout and I finish the year with another 600 hours of training and call-outs, and more finds.

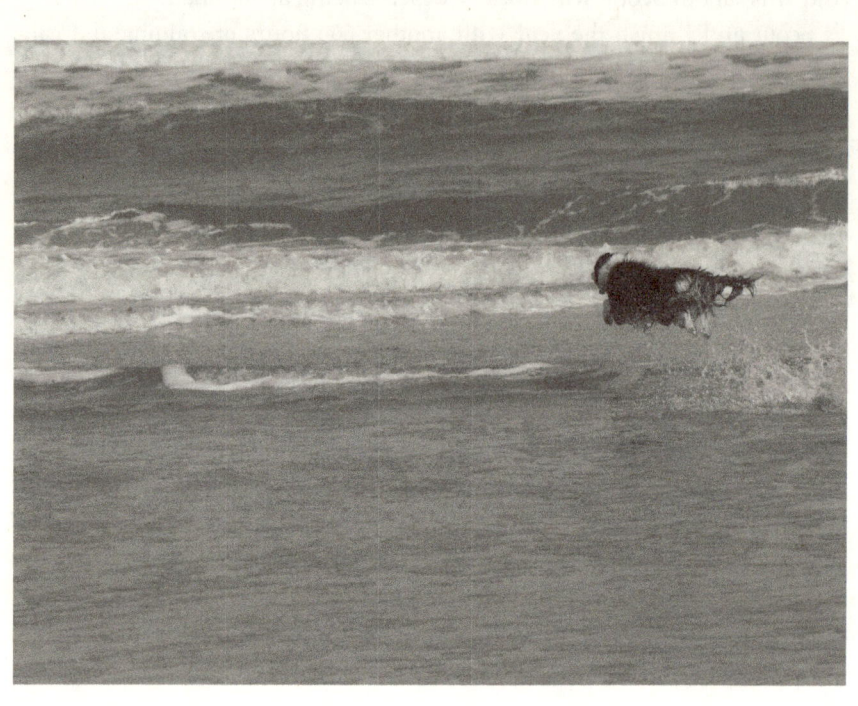

THE RESCUE

2022

The day is foul. A storm is rolling through, high winds driving hail and rain, bitterly cold. Not a day to be out. Perfect for training.

We are at a high level, very exposed with little protection from the elements that are battering the land, the leading edge of the major storm that will hit the country in a few days.

I want to look at refining my directional control to get Scout moving around more efficiently. After the disappointment of Wales had settled, I'd sat down with Steve and devised a plan of action. Our new strategy will rely on technical prowess and an advanced reading of conditions.

A long ridge forms my eastern boundary of Sir William Hill, the trig pillar top left, then turning north along to Gotherage Plantation, then on to the jumble of wall corners and stile leading down to the valley at Stoke Ford. From the stile, follow the wall bordering Eyam Moor north-east, to Rock Basin, and enclose the search area. Centre ground is humps and hollows, an outcrop, a ring cairn, public footpaths and a wind howling like a whirling dervish – by the look of the trees it's fifty miles per hour. It's the highest point, a square of flat moor, the sides running down to valleys, funnelling the wind, pulling what's behind ever faster. Pulses of rain and hail punch through, then a lull, the moor calming, then all hell breaking loose again. A handful of walkers fight their way across the moor, the forces pushing them over, the only way forward a crouching head-down hold-on-to-everything slog. I know there are two bodies here, bunkered out of the wind. I know this because I asked for that – I want to do technical work, try different scenarios, into the wind, away from the wind, see how far away

Scout detects scent and what happens to scent when it gets kicked around by a storm. One of the bodies is an old hand, the other is here for the first time.

On to the ridge, Scout settles down. I watch to see if he gets any scent dumps outside our search area. Nothing. We move along the ridge, boulders slippery with verglas. We're not high, thirty metres or so above the flat moor. But we are now the highest object, and the wind finds us an easy target, shoving me around, driving sharp hail into my face and sucking my breath out of me. It's hard going on the body; even with all my protection of winter gear and goggles, my flesh flash-freezes, searingly burns then thaws. Scout is in his element, having a happy time investigating the deluge of scents barrelling towards him, his fur swept sideways downwind, his right side sleek and smooth as he cuts across. Thirty minutes in, his nose snaps into the wind and he scrambles down the ridge on to the moor. I can see the white tip of his tail telegraphing his progress. I can't hear the bell above all the screaming. He's coming back, he's found, all his attention on me as he picks his way up, the wind pushing him into the rock as he moves. When I follow, the wind throws me around like a rag then punches me into the rock, fingers bending in ways they shouldn't as I shoot hands out for balance. I can feel my body calling for energy. It's a lovely find, the body snug in the bivvy, well out of sight. They tell me it's -12 °C windchill. I say to stay wrapped while I play with Scout.

We head back up to the ridge to carry on. Wailing banshees drag oxygen out of every cell as I battle through to the trig, shoving the negatives piling in away from me.

I figure Scout's strike was 200 metres, at least, that's the amount of ground he has cleared as we worked along the ridge. We move that far towards Gotherage Plantation and begin our return track. I discount the top-right corner, knowing Scout would have sensed anything there. It's been forty-five minutes, and I'm exhausted mentally and physically. I'm taking too long. My thinking is muddled, the gale moving from serene to anger is taking its toll, my chest heaves for air, my brain whirls around inside my hood. I lose track of my position, where we've been, the moor looking different down here to how it looks from above. I'm facing trees ahead, so I reason I must be heading that way and have cleared what is behind me and to my left.

A small group of walkers cross; I watch as they support each other, arms outstretched, gloved fingers gripping the pack in front. The wind strikes, batters them into a cube as they crab forwards. The banshees fall silent. As the angels pass, the group stands. Angered by their arrogance the wind is furious, the trees bending low, moving as one against the onslaught. I crouch with Scout and keep my eyes on the group, watch them hit the ground on all fours, heads down. Hard rain and piercing ice strafes plastic clothing and human flesh. My heart and lungs raging in complaint, Scout leans in, sticks his nose under my chin, his warm breath comforting. My brain whispers, *something is not right*.

There's a shallow dip along the wall running down to the final boundary, where the walkers are. We make sure we clear it; it's perfect for a refuge in this storm. Back at the start of the ridge, we stop. That's it, we've worked the area, and still one body to find.

I know what has happened. And where the body is. I haven't made a mistake, haven't missed Scout's indication. The body is in the corner where I decided not to go, the point where my mind and body began shutting down.

The reasons for the fail weigh heavily. We've taken shelter in the lee of rock, the air quietened; I work through what happened. I didn't go there, didn't send Scout to that top corner, because my body and mind had blown a fuse, and I couldn't muster the need. If it had been a call-out, it could have been a life lost. I'm no longer reliable. In that moment lies the end of our time as a search dog team. It's over.

How much time passes with my eyes staring into the moor, I don't know. I've travelled to a very dark place; recrimination and failure slams doors. The darkness is punctured by a cold wet nose forcing its way between my clasped hands and planting itself on my cheek. Scout's beautiful brown eyes hold me. '*It's okay, I've got you.*' 'I know,' I tell him, 'I'm glad you have.'

I want to get the body we've missed. I owe Scout that. We have never finished an exercise without finding the bodies and we won't begin now. This is our last hurrah.

The storm hits again, slicing the moor with the horizontal tracing of freezing hail and rain, firing straight through clothing, flesh and bone. I watch as a walker battles towards the wall for protection, bent at the waist, keeping their head down as they aim for the descent to Stoke Ford and, hopefully, easier times. When the ground is clear I send Scout out into the storm.

As I battle on to the moor, Scout is heading down to the stile; I figure he's got the scent of the bent-double walker. An outcrop shields my view of him, and in the screams his bell is virtually useless. Above me on the ridge a walker stands by the triangulation pillar and watches the storm over my head. I turn and push into the blast of hail and rain.

Halfway to the second body I think I hear a bark, Scout trying to find me or asking me to wait. I turn and crouch to look for him. He's heading to me, his fur sweeping around him in the blast. I can see ice forming on his feathers. I throw out my arms to gather him in, warm him. As he enters my protection, he speaks, loud, spins and heads back the way he came. I was wrong. We haven't missed the body, we haven't failed. The body was somewhere behind us. We must have been on the wrong side of the wind. That jumble of wall corners twisting the wind around, the walkers muddling the scent.

He's back, eyes on fire, the storm whipping off his body as though it isn't there. Another speak, this time jumping at me and grabbing my hand in his mouth. I pull it back in shock, only to see his tale retreating into the storm again. I half run almost falling over as I stumble over the outcrop to be met by Scout and another indication and another hand grab. No broken skin.

In front there is the wall, over that Eyam Moor. Scout is running down towards the stile. It's then I see the body in a ditch. As I approach, I launch his toy and shout praise, the wind taking the ball and my words beyond him. He pirouettes to chase them down, leaving the black mass crouching.

The body hasn't moved, no sudden spring into the air to play with Scout. I guess it's the newbie, but they are in one hell of a state. The storm hasn't been kind. Their clothes are soaking, the exposed hands look white and clammy, the whole bundle shivering. I shout my presence. The head lifts and I see it isn't the body.

It's a member of the public. Kneeling by them I ask if they are okay. The waxy white face shakes, words tumbling from thin ashen lips. I engulf them in my belay jacket, zip it tight, put dry hat and gloves on, pour hot tea to hold and sip, shove a Mars bar in their hand, tell them to eat and drink while I shield them from the wind to hold the warmth in. They have cheap summer walking gear, totally unsuited to a winter storm, sodden walking shoes and freezing extremities. I wrap my emergency shelter round us both, safer than trying to open it in the storm, and get Scout to lie between their legs, drop some treats to keep him there, let his warmth flow through to them. In the next minutes I check the pulse, a little faint and a little slow. They're overwhelmed by the weather but not resisting my help. When they begin to talk it's a little disjointed. They weren't expecting it to be this bad. They'd been out in this all day, hoping things would improve. As they'd climbed out of the valley from Stoke Ford the wind and rain had hit hard. Not knowing what to do they'd curled up. I don't mention hypothermia.

A voice shouts through the wind telling me he'd seen it all happen. Says the dog found them in a ditch. They were wet and cold and shivering.

The dog barked at them then ran away. He asks if we need help; I think we are okay, I say, and he heads down into the safety of the valley.

Finally, a smile from the casualty. As they tell me a little of their day they begin to come back into the world. We'll take a steady walk off together, take our time. I radio the rendezvous to expect us and call the unfound dogsbody out. It's slow, steady progress, Scout holding his reward toy and pathfinding the way ahead. When we arrive, others take charge warming the casualty back to being a normal live human being.

I dry Scout, his rumble growl of happiness rolling out, tell him how proud I am, how fantastic he was, settle him into bed to enjoy a chew. The unfound body appears. They were in the top corner.

I tell Alison about the day. The weather, the missed body, my fitness and mind. And Scout's find. It is, I say, his most important find. He gets lots of praise and hugs; all three dogs get sausages for tea. Over the next few days, emails arrive congratulating us on a 'proper find'. It means a lot.

Alison and I talk about the work in mountain rescue, my writing, the asbestosis, my well-being, our well-being. I know she is really upset about the prognosis of the disease. We both know what lies ahead, have researched how this ends – it isn't pleasant. We don't know how long I have. The one thing I don't want is to have her life destroyed looking after me, and I don't want to be fighting for every single breath just to exist. I can control the how and when I die. I make enquiries; £10,000, including flight, accommodation and packaging. Bargain.

Until then, what do we do? Alison says, live. Let's live life fully. Remember when you stopped drinking, you chose life rather than alcohol. Remember when you fell off that mountain, you chose to get straight back out there. Remember when it all went wrong in training, you chose to go on your own. That's why you have Scout, that's why those people he found, those you helped, their families, have a future today. Because you chose to not give in. Because you chose to live.

The hospital passes on details of support organisations, who supply a list of solicitors specialising in industrial asbestos cases. There's cost involved. The solicitor asks if I'm in a union. Not since I left the steelworks, I'm not even sure my union is still around, I say. A search for the union takes me to their present incarnation; I email, not expecting anything. They ask my solicitor to contact them; within the hour they've agreed to fund the case and made me a full union member again.

The solicitor needs statements from people I worked with, that I have not seen or heard of for almost forty years. I track some down and they agree to help and invite me to a Christmas gathering. When I get there, it's almost empty, a kid playing a machine, a table of old men chatting, a man with a dog. Walking back to the door one old man turns, and I recognise him from the steelworks. They look so old; that shocks me as it must mean I do too, but when we talk, they become the faces I used to see back in the 1980s. We are young again.

The respiratory consultant discharges me into the care of the Interstitial Lung Disease Team in Sheffield. There are several centres of specialism around the country dealing with lung diseases, including many caused by work. Sheffield's steel industry has laid a heavy hand across many lives. I'm given more tests, then see a new consultant. Alison comes, she wants to know everything.

It's bad and good news. Two CT scans show my lung function has seen a significant deterioration. The good news is I qualify for a drug that may slow down the progression of the asbestos scarring; it's expensive and not everyone can tolerate the side effects that can be very unpleasant. If I can deal with the downside it might help. It's not a cure, will not stop the disease, but the manufacturer's test data shows it can extend life eleven years on average. I say yes.

He asks a little about my background. I talk about the steelworks, the daily contact with the asbestos, the safety officer asking me to rip some off for the company to check if it was dangerous, me doing it, just to be helpful, and how I think about that a lot. My time in mountain rescue, the outdoors, the difficulty I now have getting around the hills.

Asbestos has been in use for thousands of years, the dangers first recorded in 1895, the first documented death from exposure in 1906. The material was banned in the UK in 1999, but in the 1970s and 1980s, even though the dangers were known, no one told us. A major problem with the disease is its long latency period before health issues become evident; it's taken forty years for me, about average.

The consultant talks about how the asbestos fibres floating in the air are drawn into the lungs, tiny strands and specks of dust, working their way on air currents down the trachea, through the bronchioles, catching on tissue, forming tiny rafts of material that lie across oxygen-carrying vessels, settling in the alveoli. The body's defence mechanism sees a threat, and slowly seals the asbestos from the surrounding tissue. This is the lung scarring, like the scab on a kid's knee, only this one can't be picked. The scarring seals off the alveoli, stopping the transfer of fresh oxygen into the bloodstream and waste carbon dioxide out of the blood. As well as starving my muscles of oxygen, it's also poisoning me. The lungs will gradually harden, like a bag of old cement, becoming less flexible until eventually they will cease to function.

I can feel how tense Alison is, how near she is to tears. This is the first time she has sat and someone else, someone who knows, has explained the disease. Asbestosis is usually slowly progressive, and many patients die with it, rather than of it. If it is progressive, then deaths can occur from respiratory failure, or due to the body's reduced reserve to cope with lung infections. There is also an increased risk of death from cancer due to the asbestos exposure.

He asks if we have seen the images from the CT scan? We haven't. Do we want to look? We do.

On the screen two large black masses appear. We both say, 'Oh dear.' 'That's your lungs,' he says. We travel through my lungs like some sci-fi movie, going vertically down; white tree-like branches appear. We say, 'Oh dear.' 'That's the blood vessels,' he says and continues further into the depths. Halfway down, a silver line begins to dawn on the edge of the lung, tiny silver streaks, microscopic contrails, crossing each other, shading my lungs and body, running all the way to the bottom and back up the other side. The lungs have been dipped in moonlight. 'That's the lung scarring,' he says. It's beautiful.

The antidepressants have begun to take effect, and the talking therapy is actually proving beneficial. It's like being given permission to be me. It seems I'm an introvert, hence dog handler. Who knew? Lots of things fall into place: my dislike of big groups, busy places, social functions. I prefer my own company, a very small group of friends, whom I see not too often, spending my time with Alison, Monty, Olly and Scout.

The solicitor preparing my case for compensation refers me to a medical expert. In his High Court testimony, he will say, having examined me, that he concludes the asbestosis is aggressive and he would not expect me to be alive in five years' time. He also cannot dismiss the possibility that lung cancer or mesothelioma will develop.

Time is now our currency. To spend it wisely we need to make changes, remove anything and anyone that has a negative influence on our life. That is the first step.

I cut back on commitments; no more guidebooks or magazine articles to research. I build my days around mornings of writing, afternoons of reading, culture, eating. Alison expands her culinary repertoire. I post images of food on social media. Alison adds modelling and acting to her artistic and culinary talents; Scout gets a modelling agent.

Alison knows she needs to protect herself. It's much harder for her, she has the worry of me, and the worry of what her own future holds, alone. I'm glad she's constructing her new life. I move to two sleeps a day, the first late afternoon after dinner, when I'm tired. Rested, I read in the evening, then sleep until mid-morning. It's clear I'm not going to be scaling any mountains again, so I divest myself of all my gear, giving most away.

Slowly, we find our way into a new rhythm of life. I walk with Scout, shorter distances, low level. My lung function continues to deteriorate; it's picking up speed, in two years it will have halved. On walks we seek out the interesting. Instead of pounds of kit I carry a notebook and pencil to sit and draw, and I pack treats for Scout who lies by my side to enjoy a post-snack snooze. We travel by bus and train, which Scout likes the best, as he gets lots of floor space and loads of attention. Our family life is happy and carefree. We try to remain in the present and not worry about yesterday or tomorrow. I think a lot about what Scout taught me. That you can just move on, find more enjoyable things to do and people to be with. That there is no need to hold the past or the future in the present. It turns out he's a great philosopher.

I speak to Steve regularly over the phone. We start by running down our list of ailments, doctors and hospital appointments, the stuff we suddenly can no longer do. It means a lot he's still there, still holding out the hand of friendship.

I meditate now, finding it a good way of reducing stress and easing my heart. The Interstitial Lung Disease Team refer me to Pulmonary Rehabilitaion and the Well-Being Team. I spend rehab being shoved on to the next exercise station by little old ladies who seem to be a lot fitter than me. I work on my anxiety and catastrophising with the mental health nurse, hoping to lead as normal a life as possible.

Alison and I talk a lot more, about our day, the near future. Alison looks after me, making sure my day runs smoothly, shoos away any negative influences. I consider us to be very fortunate. We've been given the priceless gift of knowing time is precious and not to be wasted.

We both gather friends around us, people who aren't afraid to live, share their own worlds with like minds. There is no striving any more, no competing to be chosen, none of that matters. Perhaps that is age; I also like to think it's what we have worked for. It feels like Alison and I are moving to the centre of our own cosmos.

Looking back, I see I've been preparing for this for years. Clearing out the debris from my life, putting little rituals in place that please me. My days are filled with the things I want to do. Putting words on paper helps me see the meaning of it all, the threads that weave through today from my childhood. I know I couldn't have got here if I had not lived in all those other worlds, that those times made the person today, brought this happiness and acceptance. I used to think life was one long line, beginning to end; now I see the path weaving through the labyrinth with all its twists and turns to the centre of a life well lived.

None of it would have been the truth of it all if it wasn't for Scout. He taught me to live.

I arrange to meet Body Paul on Loxley Common, the place and the person that helped Scout and I step out of the wilderness all those years ago. Scout hasn't seen him for some time so I'm excited to see them together. I tell Paul to bring his kit and a flask, and we'll sit and catch up near the trig pillar where he hid the night Scout found the lovers. It's a lovely spring evening, a slight chill under a clear sky, the stars abundant. Scout is off, freewheeling through the woodland, soon to return with eyes like dishes, full of excitement, to tell me he's found. When Paul pops out of his bivvy, Scout erupts with happiness, clambering all over him, covering him in kisses. We sit, Scout at his side, nosing for attention. I tell Paul he is our last find, that I would not have wanted it any other way. It's been a privilege, he says.

We have two more things to do, two last places to be. I drive to the team base and place my kit on a shelf, wander around remembering all that has happened. The rooms fill with voices and faces, Scout making his first appearance as a puppy, his first training session with the team, proudly wearing his operational jacket. They've been good years.

Scout roots around, I raid the biscuit barrel for him; we sit by the cold fire, drink tea, savour the moments we had here. I phone the team leader, tell him I can no longer continue, that it would not be safe for me or others. He thanks me and Scout for all we've done. By the time I've left there's an email to the team saying Scout and I will be missed.

We've stood down.

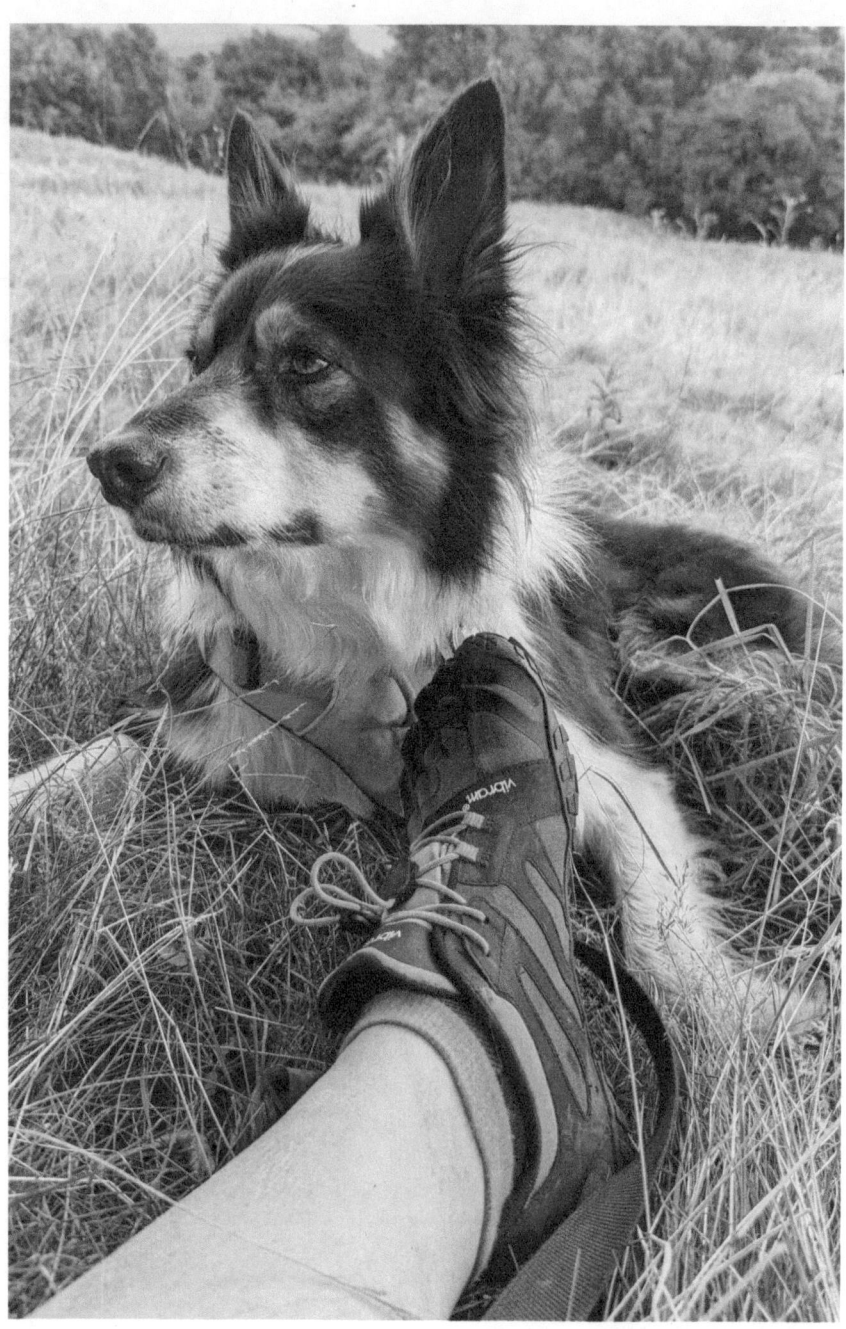

EPILOGUE

I've taken it easy up the steep path winding through the heather to Alphin Pike, pausing frequently to catch the views, and lungs full of air. Scout, higher, monitors my progress, each pause bringing his steady gaze, and if he feels it necessary, a return, his movement back down full of purposeful intent, clouds of pollen billowing around him drifting into the valley. On reaching me his eyes search deep into mine. I tell him I'm alright. His gaze remains steady. I reassure him, ruffle his hair; wisps of pollen and the heady scent of heather blossom rise into the sunlight. 'I'm alright, honest.' Words spoken softly. He leaves, reluctantly, the glances back frequent.

At the summit we rest, letting our bodies and minds settle and the wildness of the landscape restore us. I'm glad we made this our last journey.

We don't work this land now, but we are part of it. I can see the Office where we first arrived, the bridge where the dogsbody hid, the ruins where Scout found the old boys eating their sandwiches. I can hear Steve's voice booming out across the valley, 'Trust your dog.' I can see the bracken parting in waves as Scout makes his way back to me. I can see me listening to angels pass on a crisp winter day with fresh snow and a blue sky. And I can see Scout looking out from the crag, his eyes lighting up when he sees me. Our time here is held forever.

As we move out of the Wilderness, Scout pushes on to the joy he knows is ahead. When I get to him, I join him in a swim, feeling our bodies slip through the cold water that floats beneath the clouds, our limbs keeping time, smiling our happiness.

Afterwards, we lie on the heather and let the sun warm our bodies. Everything is perfect.

Here in this valley Scout taught me that yesterday and tomorrow have no hold. That it is in the moment where life happens. And the moments are held in the land.

Below us the silver thread of *Chew Brook* carves away the grains of time. And beyond, the thin grey line of *Chew Road*, sometime dirt sometime gravel sometime tar, falls from the waters in the sky above, to the waters in the valley below.

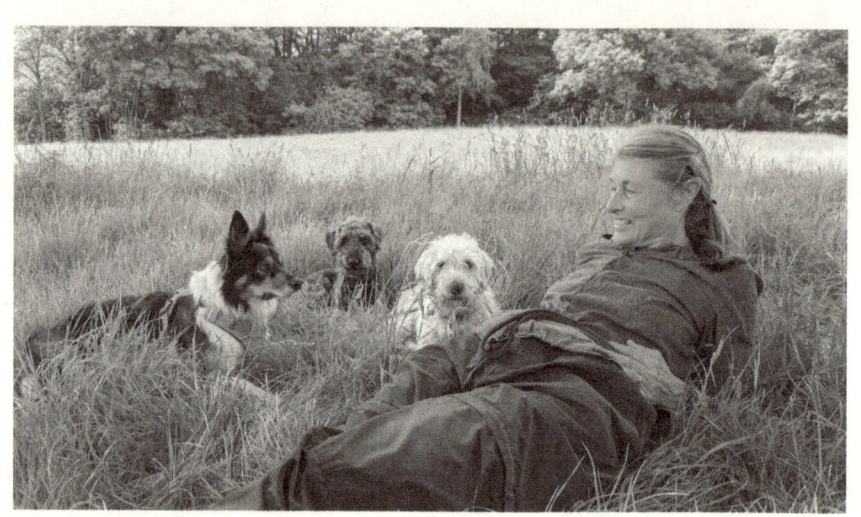

ACKNOWLEDGMENTS

'Every person that comes into our life, comes for a reason; some come to learn and others come to teach.'

Antoine de Saint-Exupéry

I have been fortunate to have many wonderful people join me in this story we call life. Some have played fleeting parts, others have walked beside me for much of the way. Some have faded into the background as life has placed space between us, only to return decades later as though they had just stepped out to feel the rain. Many knew they had made a difference to my life, but many more had no inkling what a word or gesture meant to me. As for me, I hope I have contributed – I think I have – and I hope my presence has been helpful.

As I have said, it has always been important to me to say thank you to the people who are part of my story. So, let me say thank you …

To Alison Counsell who made everything possible and taught me how to be gentle with others, and myself. You mean everything to me; I love you dearly.

To Monty and Olly who kick my bedroom door in every morning for a 'bright' start to the day.

To Stephen Ward (Wardy) who shared his knowledge, skill and trust with me. You never let me down.

To Paul Richmond, Annette Parker and Diane Earnshaw who made it possible for Scout and me to find our way out of the wilderness.

To all the people who made a difference:

The team at Vertebrate Publishing: Jon Barton, John Coefield, Kirsty Reade, Helen Parry, Jane Beagley, Lorna Brogan, Sophie Fletcher and Vicky Frost. Thank you for your support, trust and patience. To proofreader Moira Hunter.

To the lads from British Steel Corporation Rotherham works: Roger

Bostock, Ken Birch, Barry Dyson, Les Ripley and Simon Birch. Thank you for true friendship.

To the men, women and dog of Coniston Mountain Rescue Team. It all began with you.

To the real heroes – our NHS – and the respiratory specialists at the Northern General Hospital: Dr C. Burton, Dr C. Barber, nurses Sue Miller, Fiona Davis, Angela Halladay, Samantha Parkin, Helen Eyre and Samantha Hughes, and Professor J.P. Gunn – cardiology. To the people of Sheffield and Rotherham Asbestos Group (SARAG), Unite the Union, and Marion Voss of Thompsons Solicitors. To all, thank you.

To Chris Jones, Lynne and Malcolm Gibbons, Hazel White, Mike Press, Ed Douglas and Helen Mort.

To Steve Rowe, Oliver Pratt, Mick Nield, Ken Sloan, Tony Amies, David Haffenden, Mick Mellor, Mihajlo Milinkovic, Karis Hodgson, Nic and Ian Bunting, Dave Mason, Mark Williams and Sara Turner, Paul Bartram, Mike Needham, Kev Stead, John Wood, Alli Holland, Jacquie Hall, Emma Johnson, Derek and Rachel Scrimgeour, Lindsay Threlkeld and Pip, Freda and John Hill, Louise Bailey, Kirstie and Ian Martin, Claire Starkey, Jim Burgess and Midge, Joseph Massey, Granville Toyn, John Driver, Tom Mills, Ian Dredge, Julie Dignan, Denzil Broadhurst, Tomo Thompson, Hattie Earle, Katherine Aalto, Beth Anne Macdonald, Veronica Martin, Peaches Davis, Elizabeth Wainwright, Kim Krauss, Maria Benjamin, Scott Whitham, Hannah Smalley, Dale Bird, Andrew Beevers, Trish Noble, Angela and Barry Foster, David Gaines, Sarah Lister, Sally Goldsmith, Mark Richards, Sally Fawcett, Paul Weston, David Holmes, Jacqui Ní Bhroin, Johannes J. Arens, Mark Goodwin, Brian Lewis, Peter Judd, Shirley Thorpe, John Halstead, Mark Harrison, Ash Routen, Keith Wakeley, Jim Perrin, Jeff Carrol and Andrew Symonds.

Finally, and for me, most importantly, to my hill buddy, Scout. Each day you teach me about life and how to squeeze the absolute most out of each moment. You are gentle and kind, strong and fearless. You saw in me the things I never knew. I love you to bits. From my heart, thank you for finding me.

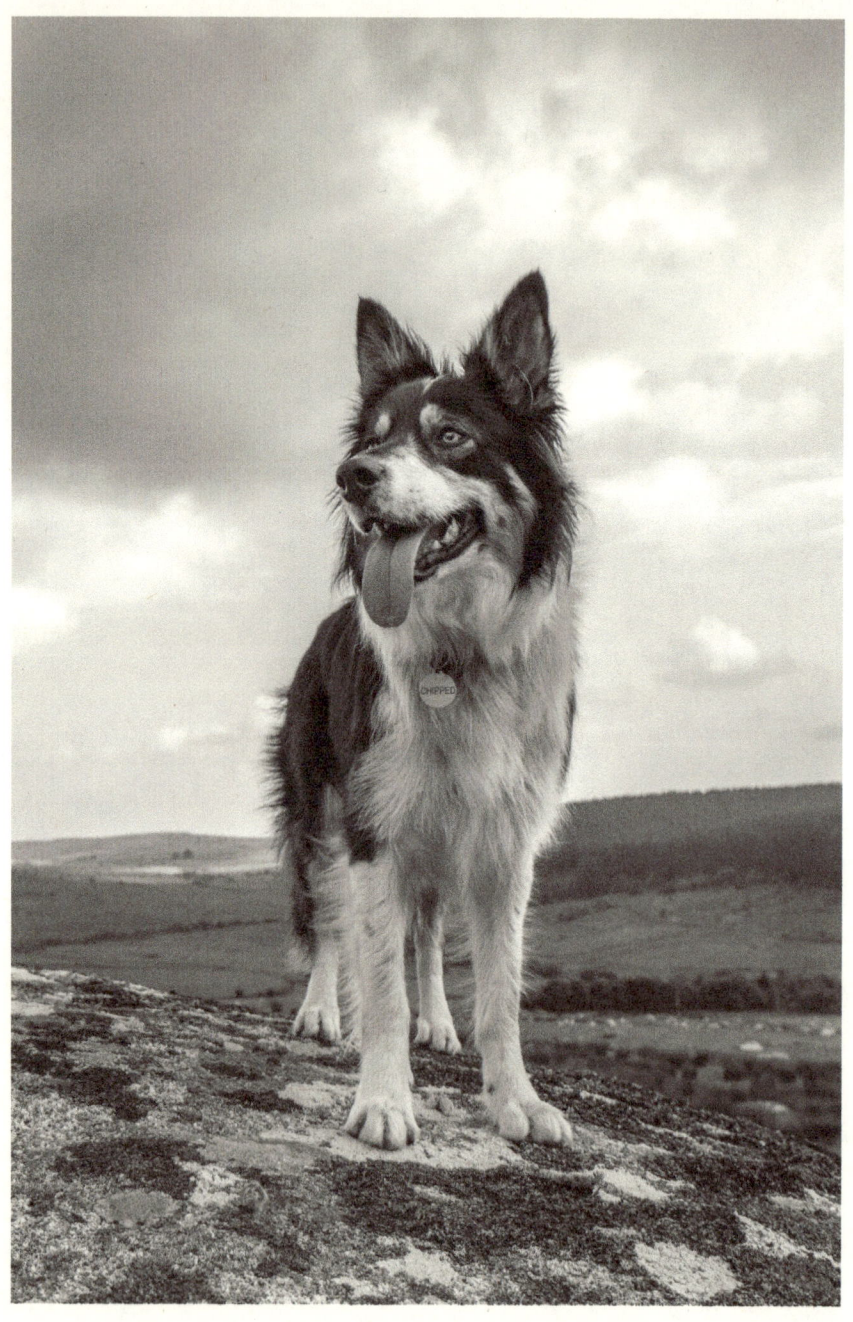